Radiology at the University of Pennsylvania

1890–1975

Radiology at the University of Pennsylvania 1890–1975

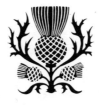

Published for the Department of Radiology
at the
University of Pennsylvania
by the University of Pennsylvania Press
Philadelphia
1981

*Published for the Department of Radiology
at the University of Pennsylvania
by the University of Pennsylvania Press.*

Library of Congress Cataloging in Publication Data

Leopold, Lynne Allen.
  Radiology at the University of Pennsylvania, 1890–
1975.

  "Special limited edition of 300 copies"—Verso t.p.
  Bibliography: p.
  1. University of Pennsylvania. Dept. of Radiology—
History. I. University of Pennsylvania. Dept. of
Radiology. II. Title.
R899.L46   1981   616.07'57'071174811   81–40557
ISBN 0–8122–7820–8   AACR2

Printed in the United States of America

Contents

CONTENTS

The Move to the Agnew Pavilion—
October 1897
[11]

The Department Under Leonard:
1896–1902
[11]

Notes
[16]

THE PANCOAST ERA, 1902–1939

The Department Under New Leadership—1902
[21]

Henry Khunrath Pancoast—Biographical Information
[22]

Growth Under Henry K. Pancoast,
1903–04
[22]

The Fourth Annual Meeting of the
American Roentgen Ray Society:
Houston Hall, University of Pennsylvania,
Philadelphia, December 9–10, 1903
[24]

The New Facility: 1904–05
[27]

The Establishment of the Philadelphia
Roentgen Ray Society—1905
[31]

Continued Expansion of Services:
1905–11
[32]

The Nation's First Professor
of Roentgenology—1911
[36]

Growth and National Recognition Before World War I
[38]

CONTENTS

CONTENTS

THE PENDERGRASS ERA, 1940–1960

CONTENTS

CONTENTS

A LOOK TOWARD THE FUTURE
Stanley Baum
[139]

Appendix: Personnel in the Department of Radiology,
Hospital of the University of Pennsylvania, 1899–1973
[143]

Bibliography
[157]

Full-Time Faculty, Department of Radiology: Hospital of the
University of Pennsylvania, 1981
[161]

Preface

Shortly after he became Chairman of the Department of Radiology in July, 1975, Stanley Baum expressed interest in a departmental history to Francis James Dallett, Archivist of the University of Pennsylvania. Mr. Dallett passed that information on to me, and I began my research in December of that year.

Dr. Baum's enthusiasm for the project and the willingness of current and former staff members to speak with me made the work possible. Eugene P. Pendergrass, M.D., was especially cooperative in answering my questions and passing along materials from his files. Their encouragement, plus that of Robert M. Stein, Associate Dean of the School of Medicine, then Department Administrator, permitted me to investigate the department's history at length.

I presented two lectures to the department's staff on my research: "The Department before World War I" on May 27, 1976, and "The Pendergrass Era" on September 22, 1976.

A first draft of the manuscript covering the period through Dr. Pendergrass's chairmanship was completed in the fall of 1976, but it has taken me until now to revise and complete the work. My full-time position as an Assistant Curator at Independence National Historical Park has kept me busy, and I would not have been able to complete the project yet, were it not for the professional support and understanding of my supervisor, John C. Milley, Chief, Division of Museum Operations.

My training as a social scientist provided the tools necessary to write the history of the department, but not the technical expertise which was needed periodically. I am grateful to John

Hale, Radiological Physicist, and others, who took the time to clarify technical matters for me.

With the assistance of all those listed in the following Acknowledgments, however, the responsibility for errors is mine alone.

Philadelphia   Lynne Allen Leopold
November, 1978

Acknowledgments

One of the most enjoyable aspects of this project has been the opportunity to talk about the history of the department with both former and present staff members and consultants. Their assistance has proven invaluable in the compilation of information, and their personal insights and anecdotes add immeasurably to the text. My special thanks go to Robert P. Barden, M.D., Larissa T. Bilaniuk, M.D., Edward M. DeYoung, M.D., Adele K. Friedman, M.D., Philip J. Hodes, M.D., David E. Kuhl, M.D., Wallace T. Miller, M.D., Mark M. Mishkin, M.D., and S. Reid Warren, Sc.D.

Other members of the staff of the Department of Radiology have also generously aided me in this project. I am particularly appreciative for the assistance provided by George F. Brady, Betty Lou Ditz, Sandra A. Girifalco, Jessica M. Hullings, Margaret Joan McKee, Gary A. Pfaff, Carol J. Reynolds, and Charles D. White. Bette Schweiker, of the hospital's Administration Department, was exceedingly helpful and patient as I photocopied the entire set of *Annual Reports of the Board of Managers*.

Many individuals at research institutions throughout Philadelphia kindly assisted me with my work. I wish especially to thank Roy E. Goodman, Reference Librarian at The American Philosophical Society, Ellen G. Gartrell, Elizabeth M. Moyer and the reference librarians at The College of Physicians of Philadelphia, Stephanie A. Morris, and Francis James Dallett, and the entire staff of the University of Pennsylvania Archives and Records Center.

My most heartfelt thanks go to John Hale, Ph.D., Radiological Physicist in the department, and Eugene Percival Pendergrass,

ACKNOWLEDGMENTS

M.D., Emeritus Professor and Chief. Dr. Hale edited the first draft of the manuscript for technical errors and style, and his input was extremely valuable. Dr. Pendergrass spent many, many hours telling me about the sixty years he spent in the department, and was always willing to answer my questions.

Very special thanks also go to my friend and associate, Marilyn Kralik, and to my special friend, Daniel J. Sharp, who spent countless hours editing and proofreading the manuscript.

Without the help of these and countless other individuals, this history could not have been written. Again, thank you!

EARLY YEARS
1890–1902

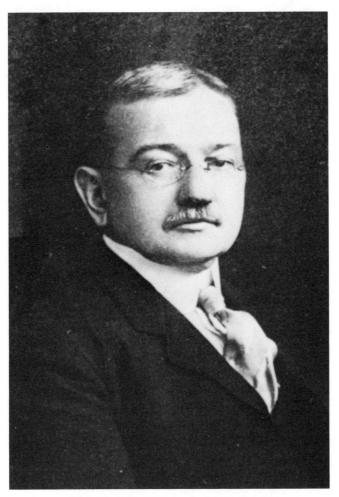

Charles Lester Leonard, 1896–1902

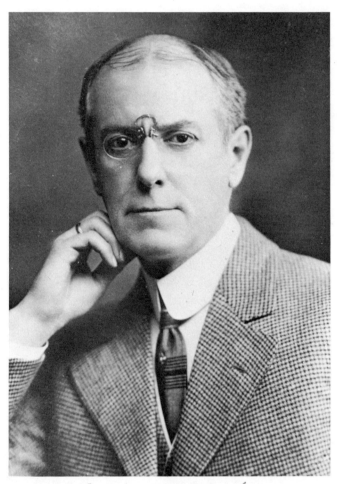

Arthur Willis Goodspeed, 1884–1931

Arthur Willis Goodspeed: Physics and Photography

Arthur Willis Goodspeed showed an aptitude for the physical sciences early in his life and while a student at Harvard University was encouraged to pursue this interest. He graduated *summa cum laude* from Harvard in 1884, with highest honors in physics, and after graduation accepted the position as Assistant in Physics at Pennsylvania. Working with George Frederick Barker, an experienced physicist and brillant lecturer whose reputation was international, Goodspeed was also able to pursue graduate work in the University's newly established Graduate School.[1]

Goodspeed came to Philadelphia the summer that Eadweard Muybridge was conducting his well-known investigations in animal locomotion on the Pennsylvania campus. The studies were sponsored by the University, and Dr. Barker served as a member of the Muybridge Commission, appointed by the Provost, to oversee the project; the young physicist, Goodspeed, was therefore involved in these experiments as soon as he arrived. It is probable that he was involved in Muybridge's later work as well, and may have helped to design an electrical device used during the work on human locomotion which released the shutters on a series of cameras in automatic sequence.[2] These experiences were undoubtedly responsible for stimulating this interest in the scientific aspects of photography, if, in fact, his interest did not originate from these experiments.[3]

Goodspeed was named an Instructor in 1885 and an Assistant Professor in 1889 when he received his doctoral degree, the first degree conferred by the new Graduate School.[4] In the fall of 1889 he began a series of experiments with W. N. Jennings, a Philadelphian who wished to make use of the facilities in the University's Physics Department. The two men spent several years photographing electric sparks produced by various pieces of apparatus and comparing them to Jennings's previous photographs of lightning. In the process they produced some startling exposures which remained unexplained until the publication of Röntgen's communications.[5]

The Accidental, Unrecognized Production of X-Rays at Pennsylvania—1890

Goodspeed and Jennings spent the evening of February 22, 1890, in the University's physics lecture room photographing the brush from a large induction machine, as well as coins and brass weights which were sparked using an induction coil. After completing these experiments Dr. Goodspeed opened a cabinet to show Jennings the laboratory's collection of Crookes tubes and exhausted one to show him the attractive colors produced by the vacuum. Following this diversion Jennings packed the photographic plates exposed during the evening and departed.

Later, while analyzing the plates from the evening's work, Jennings noticed that several plates that had not been exposed directly, but which were developed with the exposed ones, appeared fogged. The image of a mysterious disc appeared on one of the fogged plates, and the character of its impression was entirely different from that of those exposed in the normal manner. These unusual results were soon forgotten, however, and stored with the records of the other early experiments.

Early in February, 1896, following the announcement of Röntgen's discovery, Goodspeed and Jennings consulted their old records to determine whether they had ever exposed a plate completely covered by a plate holder and came across the notes from the evening in February, 1890. Hypothesizing that the shadow picture of the disc actually showed one of the coins exposed during the viewing of the Crookes tube, the experiments were repeated—with identical results. Speaking before the American Philosophical Society on February 21, 1896, Dr. Goodspeed related:

Now, gentlemen, we wish it clearly understood that we claim no credit whatever for what seems to have been a most interesting accident, yet the evidence seems quite convincing that the *first* Röntgen shadow picture was really produced almost exactly six years ago to-night, in the physical lecture room of the University of Pennsylvania.[6]

X-Ray Production in the Department of Physics— February, 1896

Soon after the announcement of Röntgen's discovery Goodspeed and his associates began to experiment with the available apparatus in the University's Physical Laboratory. They lacked a second induction coil as described by Röntgen, and were initially skeptical about the probability for success, but found that a simpler arrangement of apparatus, joining the tube to the secondary current of the first coil, would work as well. On February 5th a twenty minute exposure of a small slip of glass, a piece of sheet lead and a wedge of wood produced the first successful result. This experiment was immediately followed by an exposure of the skeleton of a human hand.[7]

In early February Goodspeed began working with John Carbutt, and their collaboration produced the first plate especially designed for X-rays. This new plate was considerably more sensitive than regular photographic plates, and when it was first tested at the Maternity Hospital in Philadelphia on February 11th, the length of exposure was decreased from over one hour to only twenty minutes.[8] Dr. H. W. Cattell, a Philadelphia physician, discussed the new discovery when he spoke before the Pathological Society in Philadelphia on February 13th[9]; most likely Goodspeed also made the exposures illustrating malformation of the hands and fingers which Cattell used in his presentation.[10] Throughout the first weeks of experimentation, in fact, physicists rather than physicians were most actively involved in the development of the field because they had ready access to the necessary apparatus.

Goodspeed's detailed presentation on the roentgen rays on February 21st before the American Philosophical Society, Philadelphia's learned scientific community, included a demonstration of his apparatus, and the fact that he transported this equipment to the meeting indicated the immediate, widespread interest created by the discovery. He outlined the historical developments preceding the production of roentgen rays, detailed his work at the University, and showed a number of slides illustrating a variety of techniques and possible uses for the X-ray. The slides included plates whose exposure time varied from a few to as many as forty-five minutes, and plates especially treated with a fluorescent material to increase their sensitivity. The exposures

included human and mouse skeletal views, a series using dia-
monds to determine the potential for reflection or refraction of
the rays, and a series to detect structural flaws in small pieces of
metal.[11]

The University's Physical Laboratory was only one of several
locations in the city where experiments were being conducted
with roentgen rays, and following Dr. Goodspeed's presentation
several other gentlemen spoke of their experiences and suggested
possible applications for the technique. Of particular interest
were the comments of Edwin J. Houston, Professor of Physics at
the Franklin Institute (who had had results similar to those of Dr.
Goodspeed's early experiments when he produced, but did not
recognize, roentgen rays while working at Central High School),
and those of John Carbutt (who postulated the development of
thin celluloid plates that would obtain better views of areas like
the elbow and shoulder).[12]

The discussion presented a clear view of the virtually limitless
possibilities for the development of X-ray techniques. From this
early date, their application to surgery and medicine was of para-
mount importance.

The Introduction of X-Rays
into Medical Use at Pennsylvania

Dr. Goodspeed's techniques were well developed by the time he
presented his paper to the American Philosophical Society, and
in late February or early March the roentgen ray procedure was
first used on patients at the University. In the early months patients were sent to Dr. Goodspeed's laboratory, a short distance
from the hospital buildings, and it was there that he made the
exposures using his apparatus.

J. William White, Professor of Clinical Surgery and Chief of
the Department of Surgery, was primarily responsible for the
introduction of this new procedure. The earliest medical X-rays
were taken of fractures or related injuries involving the extremities—areas which were easily accessible, shallow enough to require relatively brief exposures, and normally treated by members of the surgical staff. In the first written communication
outlining the application of the new procedure at University Hos-

pital, however, White discussed the most unusual case to date, the utilization of an X-ray exposure to locate a foreign object within a human body.[13]

Writing in the *University Medical Magazine* in June, 1896, Dr. White described a young child who came to the hospital in May unable to keep down any solid food and complaining of a pain in her throat. She had been unable to eat for some time, and, as she became more seriously ill, was actually beginning to starve. The skiagraph exposure showed a toy jack lodged in her esophagus, and permitted a rapid and precise decision concerning the best possible surgical procedure. Dr. White's enthusiastic support for this new procedure was clearly outlined in his conclusion to the case's discussion:

I have been much impressed by the practical importance of the Röntgen ray process in surgery, but in no instance more than in this, where, in a case in which every hour had become valuable and every effort at exploration dangerous, it substituted accuracy and promptness for otherwise unavoidable uncertainty and delay.[14]

At Pennsylvania, as elsewhere, the application of the roentgen ray process was initially almost exclusively limited to surgical procedures, but gradually it became utilized for general diagnoses as well. A particularly important paper, relating the process and detailing case histories, was written by Drs. White, Goodspeed, and Charles Lester Leonard, a young associate of White's, during the summer of 1896. Its publication in August served as a clear indication of the support for, and acceptance of, the new procedure.[15]

This clinical paper suggested general areas for application of the new process, specifically: to locate foreign bodies imbedded in tissue or located in certain organs or viscera, to analyze fractures and dislocations without further disturbing the sensitive area, and to discern deformities, primarily those of a skeletal nature. The paper highlighted fifteen cases in which the procedure had been used and included detailed photographic documentation of the various conditions. From the outset, the authors stressed their strong commitment to the rapid incorporation of this discovery into medicine: "The Röntgen method is, of course, in its infancy. It has, however, already reached a degree of usefulness that makes it obvious that the necessary apparatus will be an essential part of the surgical outfit of all hospitals and will be employed constantly in a variety of cases."[16]

[7]

This August publication was particularly important for two reasons: it was the first formal introduction of Charles Lester Leonard, and it spoke in optimistic terms of the many possible applications of the process for diagnostic work in medicine, as well as surgery. Within a short period of time Leonard was to assume primary responsibility for X-ray work at University Hospital, and his personal interest in gallstones and other forms of calculi was clearly expressed even at this time:

No practical results have yet been obtained in the discovery of these forms of calculi, but it seems within bounds to expect that after we become more familiar with the shadows cast by the normal viscera and the normal skeleton, we may be able to distinguish gallstones from malignant disease involving the ducts; may locate or exclude renal calculi in doubtful cases . . . [17]

The acceptance and utilization of the roentgen ray procedure in the work of many departments in the hospital was firmly established by early 1897. Opthalmologists and laryngologists used skiagraphy to locate foreign bodies, internists used it for diagnosis of disease growths and general diagnosis, as well as to view the internal organs, and surgeons used it as a precision tool to augment their procedures, both before surgery as an investigative aid and following surgery to determine success or failure.[18] Even more importantly, Dr. Leonard's work in a room in the William Pepper Clinical Laboratory established the operation's independence from the surgical staff.

Charles Lester Leonard, M.D.—Early Years

Charles Lester Leonard was born in Massachusetts in 1861, but grew up in Philadelphia. He graduated from the University of Pennsylvania in 1885 with a Bachelor of Arts Degree, and graduated from Harvard University in 1886 with a second undergraduate degree. He returned to Philadelphia to enter the University's School of Medicine, graduating in the class of 1889, and by the early 1890s was involved in his career work at the University: teaching and practicing medicine and investigating a variety of research projects.

Leonard was interested in photography while a student in the 1880s and was the subject in at least one series of photographs

[8]

in Eadweard Muybridge's experiments on human locomotion, in the group entitled "Man Running."[19] He became interested in microscopy and microphotography as his studies progressed, and after graduating from medical school spent time in Europe observing various techniques. Leonard returned to the University in the fall of 1891 to continue his studies in microscopy, and designed an electrically-operated lens shutter which enabled him to photograph various stages in the life cycle of microorganisms. He received a Master of Arts Degree in 1892 while serving as an Assistant Instructor in Clinical Surgery on the faculty of the School of Medicine.

Leonard continued his teaching and research work and was given space in the new William Pepper Clinical Laboratory, adjoining the hospital, when it was opened in 1895. His combined interest in photography and work in surgery under J. William White led to a natural inquisitiveness about the new roentgen ray process, and when a separate skiagraphy service was established in the Pepper Laboratory, he was chosen to run it.[20]

X-Ray Laboratories in the William Pepper Clinical Laboratory and the Department of Clinical Surgery

The roentgen ray process was accepted so quickly at University Hospital that in a few months it became inconvenient to transport patients outside the hospital complex to Dr. Goodspeed's laboratory. By September, 1896, Dr. Leonard had been given a small room on an upper floor of the William Pepper Clinical Laboratory, near his own research area, and was operating a skiagraphy service for the entire hospital community. Shortly thereafter a second roentgen plant was installed, this one in the Department of Clinical Surgery at the hospital.[21] Unlike Leonard's operation, however, this second plant was apparently used almost exclusively as a teaching resource by Dr. White: "It has been a source of great satisfaction to Dr. White in teaching and of otherwise unattainable instruction to the students."[22]

An extant photograph provides detailed information about Dr. Leonard's installation in the Pepper Laboratory, clearly showing the simplicity of its arrangement. The roentgen ray plant was

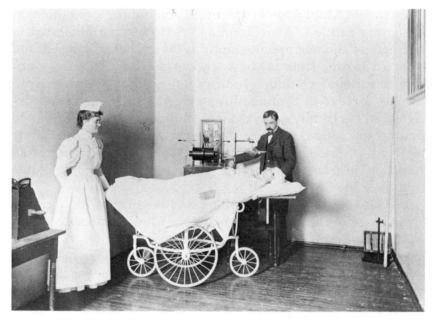

*Dr. Charles Leonard, nurse, and patient in the skiagraphy
facilities, William Pepper Clinical Laboratory, 1896*

located in a single, high-ceilinged room, with minimal equipment
and furniture. Dr. Leonard appears attending a male patient on
a litter, while Mrs. McNally, later head nurse in the Men's Surgical Ward, stands nearby, although during a routine procedure a
nurse would have been present only when the doctor was examining a female patient. The apparatus included a specialized
X-ray tube, probably designed by Edison, suspended over the
patient from a regular lab stand, since there was no roentgen ray
table in this facility. Other equipment included a 7-inch Queen
coil, powered by twenty-volt storage cells, and a mechanical
spring interrupter. There was also a fair-sized, hand-held fluoroscope, but since Dr. Leonard was never very fond of the procedure the instrument was probably used more often to test the
apparatus, to determine whether or not rays were being produced, than for fluoroscopy.[23]

The Move to the Agnew Pavilion—October, 1897

The operation of the roentgen ray apparatus in the Pepper Laboratory, although somewhat more convenient than the earlier arrangement, still provided transportation difficulties for patients. Since the operation required only minimal space, a small area was found in October, 1897, and Dr. Leonard and the entire operation moved. The hospital installed the apparatus in the new Agnew Memorial Pavilion, a decision made, however, long after building designs had been completed.

The new area was partitioned off from the waiting room of the surgical dispensary, and became a room approximately ten by twenty feet in size, with a single door and small windows high in the wall.[24] The importance of physically installing the apparatus in a main hospital building was stressed during the dedication of the new wing: ". . . laboratories, photography and Röntgen ray appliances, etc., add to the precise and scientific requirements of the day."[25]

Dr. Leonard was given a tiny room two floors above the apparatus, underneath the surgical amphitheatre, to serve as his darkroom. The space was so small that the developer could barely turn around, and because so much room was occupied by the sink a visitor or student could not observe the developing of plates. A few years later Dr. Leonard was given a larger darkroom, but the single examining room was all the working space he had for skiagraphy while at the University. These cramped quarters caused difficulties in an otherwise routine examining schedule, and would have been grossly overtaxed as a teaching facility were it not for Dr. White's installation.

The Department Under Leonard: 1896–1902

Although Charles Lester Leonard had operated the roentgen ray apparatus as an official hospital activity ever since its location in the William Pepper Clinical Laboratory, he did not use a title publically until the spring of 1898. Writing in the *Annals of Ophthalmology* in April, he was listed as "Skiagrapher to the University Hospital," the title which he retained throughout his work there.[26] Recognition of this new field of study was first accorded by the School of Medicine in the *University Catalog* for the 1898–99 academic year, under the Department of Surgery, where Leonard was listed as "Instructor in Skiagraphy," and "Assistant Instructor in Clinical Surgery"[27]; however, another faculty listing for skiagraphy did not appear until the 1903–04 *Catalog,* and Leonard was not listed as Skiagrapher in a hospital publication until the *Annual Report of the Board of Managers* for 1899.[28]

The rapid incorporation of roentgenographic procedures in many departments at University Hospital suggests a sizeable patient load, yet this was not actually the case. The first figures available, for the year 1900, indicate that Dr. Leonard saw a total of 100 patients, including sixty-nine ward patients, fourteen outpatients, ten private hospital patients, four private out-patients, and three students.[29] Considerably more than 100 exposures would have been made during the year, however, and many exposures would have lasted up to several minutes each, since the pelvis and abdomen were investigated most frequently. Because he was working alone, a fair portion of Dr. Leonard's nonteaching time was involved in preparing each patient and caring for apparatus. Patients for his final full year at the hospital, 1901, numbered 141, and the breakdown of patient categories, as well as the areas of the body examined, closely paralleled the figures from the previous year.[30]

Occasional references to apparatus during this period indicate the introduction of some new equipment to the department's operation, but there was no concerted effort to expand the services offered by the department or the physical plant in which it operated. Dr. Leonard was using self-regulating X-ray tubes by 1898, an especially important technological advance since they had ". . . made it possible to obtain a relative measurement of the vacuum employed, and to repeat at will exposures with equal vacua."[31] Leonard was also concerned with the utility of the fluoroscope, and although relatively unimpressed with its reliability in detecting accurate detail, he did recommend it for procedures such as adjusting fractures, particularly when a permanent exposure could be made later to verify the final position.[32]

Dr. J. William White presented the department with a Leeds and Northrup coil in 1899, a model which proved to be relatively portable and helped alleviate some of the difficulties caused by the narrower-than-a-bed entryway into the department's single room. The coil produced a spark somewhat heavier than earlier apparatus, and operated on a twenty volt primary circuit, supplied by a motor generator which, with proper conditions, transformed the 110 volt hospital potential into twenty volts.[33]

Cooperation among Philadelphia's physicians and scientists commenced as soon as experimentation was begun, and as one of the first skiagraphers in the city, Leonard was asked to assist in the introduction of roentgen ray apparatus at Philadelphia General Hospital in 1899. George E. Pfahler, a young physician on their staff, was asked to operate the equipment, and Leonard provided valuable insight into matters of installation and technique. He was able to persuade Pfahler to use the Queen and Company Sayen self-regulating tube, which was developed in Philadelphia and proved so successful in his own work.[34]

In addition to his clinical and teaching responsibilities, Charles Lester Leonard spent a considerable amount of time doing research and publishing the results of his clinical and research analyses. These works reveal that he considered the roentgen ray procedure an important diagnostic tool. He detailed its use in the location of foreign bodies in the eye and its practicality for the determination of fractures, and stressed the utility of the fluoroscope in a number of articles. His most extensive and sophisticated work was in the field of calculus diagnosis, and beginning in 1898 he devoted as much time as possible to this project.

Leonard was the first roentgenologist to identify kidney stones in a skiagraph, a possibility which he had foreseen as early as the summer of 1896. Several technical obstacles complicated the diagnosis of calculus nephritis, principally the fact that kidneys lie deep inside the body cavity and stones vary considerably in their individual opaqueness; however, the development of the self-regulating tube enabled the roentgenologist to duplicate conditions time and time again, and after making exposures of the organs and completing follow-up surgery, Leonard was able to delineate criteria to analyze future exposures. His initial communication on this subject, in *The Philadelphia Medical Journal* of August, 1898, continued to explain:

The absolute conditions essential to the detection of calculi in the kidney have been determined and proved repeatedly by positive clinical

[13]

evidence, so that it is certain that under these known conditions a renal calculus must be detected, and that the absence of the shadow of a calculus, in a negative showing certain definite details, is conclusive evidence of the non-existence of all calculi in that region.[35]

This early publication was only the beginning of a long series of important papers on calculus which he continued to write throughout most of the remainder of his life, and for this work Leonard is recognized as one of the most important American contributors to work on the gastrointestinal tract.[36]

Some of Leonard's patients with calculus nephritis were examined at University Hospital, but a great many were private patients whom he saw during his morning office hours in his office in center city Philadelphia. As his reputation spread he became more and more involved in the diagnosis of calculi, although at the same time he also expanded his general roentgenologic work, accepting the position of Demonstrator in Roentgen-Ray Diagnosis at the Philadelphia Polyclinic Laboratories.[37] Eventually he became Director of the program there as well as at Methodist Episcopal Hospital.[38] To further complicate this increase in his outside responsibilities, not to mention his teaching and clinical responsibilities at the University, Leonard's health was failing as a result of overexposure to X-rays.

Charles Lester Leonard, like nearly all of the pioneers of American roentgenology, suffered severely from X-ray burns. He first mentioned this problem in June, 1897, when he spoke to the Section on Practice of Medicine of the American Medical Association, indicating that the burns were caused by induced electric currents in the patient's tissues, rather than by the X-rays themselves. Leonard, along with a great many other roentgenologists, thought that the solution to the problem was to provide a means for grounding the electrical current. For some time the placement of a sheet of aluminum between the patient and the tube, with a wire leading to the floor to ground the metal, was thought to prevent the X-ray burn while still allowing the ray's beneficial penetrating force to be transmitted.[39]

Leonard's theories about the properties of the X-ray eventually changed, quite likely as the result of his continued problem with burns on his hands. At the Fourth Annual Meeting of the American Roentgen Ray Society in 1903, he described the simple form of protection he had devised: a pasteboard box covered with lead surrounding the X-ray tube to prevent secondary rays from

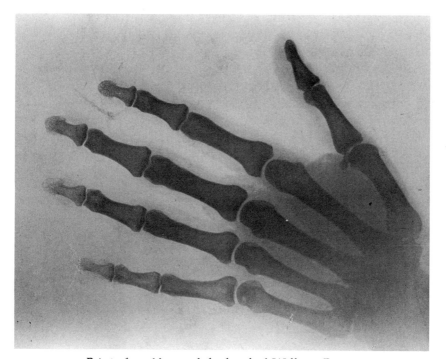

Print of an X-ray of the hand of William Pepper,
Dean of the School of Medicine, c. 1900

spreading throughout the room. He also outlined the treatments he had used to provide relief of his condition, concluding: "We all have used some kind of treatment, and I think we ought to tell each other just what we have done, so that these various remedies that have been used may be tried by others, perhaps with some success."[40]

Charles Lester Leonard left University Hospital in September, 1902, and although his other responsibilities were undoubtedly a consideration, the severity of the burns on his hands must have played a role in his departure. Skepticism and fear still surrounded the roentgen ray process, and Dr. Leonard's disability could only have served to increase the uncertainty felt by the hospital's patients. He continued to work steadily until a few years before his death in 1913, but in that period cancer spread from his hand, where a single finger had been amputated, throughout his entire body. The subsequent amputation of his hand, forearm and finally the upper arm at the shoulder joint could do nothing to stop the spread of the disease. Continually

[15]

aware of the dangers involved in X-ray work, he wrote several papers cautioning his fellow workers.[41]

The contributions of Charles Lester Leonard to the evolution of the Department of Roentgenology at University Hospital, and to the specialty of roentgenology as a whole, are of vital importance. He published twenty-nine articles while working at the University and a great many more after his departure, and his reputation in the diagnosis of calculi was international. He served as the American representative to a number of European conferences,[42] and remained a vital force in the Philadelphia roentgenologic community. In 1905 he invited the city's roentgenologists to his office for a meeting, and under his guidance a dozen physicians and scientists founded the Philadelphia Roentgen Ray Society; he served as its permanent secretary until his death.[43]

The success Leonard achieved at University Hospital, working in cramped spaces with minimal equipment, set the precedent for the department's future. With limited resources he built a sturdy foundation upon which his successors would nurture and expand the department which he had begun.

NOTES

1. Horace C. Richards, "Arthur Willis Goodspeed: An Obituary," *The American Philosophical Society Yearbook, 1943* (Philadelphia: 1944), p. 384.

2. Gordon Hendricks, *Eadweard Muybridge: The Father of the Motion Picture* (New York: Grossman Publishers, 1975), p. 157.

3. Richards, "Arthur Willis Goodspeed," p. 385.

4. Edward P. Cheyney, *History of the University of Pennsylvania, 1740–1940* (Philadelphia: University of Pennsylvania Press, 1940), pp. 297–98.

5. Arthur W. Goodspeed, "Remarks made at the Demonstration of the Röntgen Ray, at Stated Meeting, February 21, 1896," *Proceedings of the American Philosophical Society,* **35**, No. 150 (1896): 24.

6. *Ibid.*

7. *Ibid.,* p. 21.

8. Arthur W. Fuchs, "Radiographic Recording Media and Screens," in *The Science of Radiology,* ed. Otto Glasser (Springfield, Illinois: Charles C. Thomas, 1933), pp. 101–102.

9. William A. Evans, "American Pioneers in Radiology," in *The Science of Radiology,* ed. Otto Glasser (Springfield, Illinois: Charles C. Thomas, 1933), p. 26.

10. Goodspeed, "Remarks," p. 21.

11. *Ibid.*

12. *Ibid.*

13. J. William White, "A Foreign Body in the Esophagus Detected and Located by Röntgen Rays," *University Medical Magazine* 8 (1896): 710–15.

14. *Ibid.*, p. 715.

15. J. William White, Arthur W. Goodspeed, and Charles L. Leonard, "Cases Illustrative of the Practical Application of the Röntgen Rays in Surgery," *American Journal of the Medical Sciences,* 112, No. 2 (1896): 125–47.

16. *Ibid.*, p. 125.

17. *Ibid.*, p. 126.

18. "Skiagraphy in Medicine and Surgery: An Editorial," *University Medical Magazine* 9 (1897): 360–62.

19. Hendricks, "Eadweard Muybridge," p. 180.

20. Percy Brown, *American Martyrs to Science through the Roentgen Rays* (Springfield, Illinois: Charles C. Thomas, 1936), p. 113.

21. "The Extension of the Practical Application of the Röntgen Rays: An Editorial," *University Medical Magazine* 8 (1896): 967.

22. "Skiagraphy in Medicine," p. 361.

23. Henry K. Pancoast, "Reminiscences of a Radiologist," *American Journal of Roentgenology and Radium Therapy,* 39, No. 2 (1938): 171.

24. *Ibid.*

25. DeForest Willard, "History and Description of the D. Haynes Agnew Memorial Pavilion of the University Hospital," in *The Opening of the Agnew Wing at the Hospital of the University of Pennsylvania, October 15, 1897* (Philadelphia: J. B. Lippincott Company, 1897), p. 16.

26. Charles L. Leonard, "Methods of Precision in Locating Foreign Bodies in the Head by Means of the Roentgen Rays, with Special Reference to Foreign Bodies in the Eye," *Annals of Opthamology* 7, No. 2 (1898): 161.

27. *Catalogue of the University of Pennsylvania, Fasciculus of the Department of Medicine* (1898–99), p. 237.

28. Hospital of the University of Pennsylvania, *Annual Report of the Board of Managers* (31 December 1899), p. 7.

29. Hospital of the University of Pennsylvania, *Annual Report of the Board of Managers* (31 December 1900), p. 97.

30. Hospital of the University of Pennsylvania, *Annual Report of the Board of Managers* (31 December 1901), p. 102.

31. Charles L. Leonard, "The Diagnosis of Calculus Nephritis by Means of the Roentgen Rays," *Philadelphia Medical Journal* II, No. 8 (1898): 389.

32. Charles L. Leonard, "The Influence of the X-ray Method of Diagnosis upon the Treatment of Fractures," *Therapeutic Gazette* 14 (1898): 178.

33. Pancoast, "Reminiscences," p. 171.

34. George E. Pfahler, "The Early History of Roentgenology in Philadelphia: The History of the Philadelphia Roentgen Ray Society, Part I: 1899–1920," *American Journal of Roentgenology, Radium Therapy and Nuclear Medicine,* **75**, No. 1 (1956): 16.

35. Leonard, "Calculus Nephritis," p. 389.

36. George W. Holmes, "American Radiology: Its Contributions to the Diagnosis and Treatment of Disease," *Journal of the American Medical Association* **135**, No. 6 (1947): 327–30.

37. Charles L. Leonard, "A Double Focus X-ray Tube for the Accurate Localization by Fluoroscope or Photographic Plate of Foreign Bodies," *American X-ray Journal* **5** (1899): 659.

38. Brown, "American Martyrs," p. 117.

39. Charles L. Leonard, "The Application of the Roentgen Rays to Medical Diagnosis," *Journal of the American Medical Association* **29** (1897): 1158.

40. *Transactions of the Fourth Annual Meeting of the American Roentgen Ray Society, December 9–10, 1903* (Philadelphia: 1904), pp. 253–54.

41. Brown, "American Martyrs," p. 121.

42. *Ibid.*, p. 122.

43. Pfahler, "Early History of Roentgenology," pp. 14–22.

THE PANCOAST ERA
1902–1939

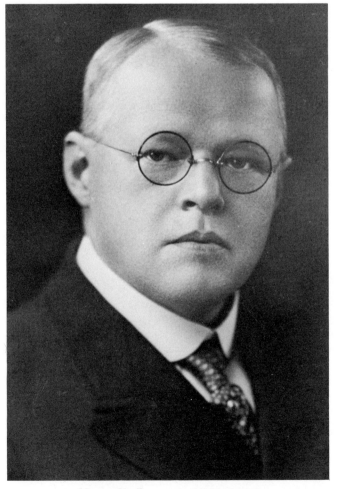

Henry K. Pancoast, 1903–1937

The Department Under New Leadership—1902

By May, 1902, J. William White, Chief of the Department of Surgery, was looking for someone to replace Dr. Leonard and operate the Roentgen Ray Department, a subdivision of the Department of Surgery. He turned to a young surgeon on his staff, and offered the position of Skiagrapher to Henry Khunrath Pancoast should Dr. Leonard definitely decide to leave the hospital.[1] Meanwhile White encouraged Pancoast to speak with Arthur Goodspeed about the basics of the X-ray phenomenon as training for his new work.[2]

Pancoast decided to accept the position, and the hospital staff was very pleased with his leadership of the department. Only a few months after he assumed his new responsibilities, the President of the Board of Managers commended his work, saying: "The X-Ray Department has been materially improved in its usefulness, and is now extensively used in Skiagraphy and Therapeutic work." Faced with severe limitations in space and equipment, Pancoast did manage to make substantial advances in the department's operation during the final months of 1902, and as he clearly stated: "The hospital could not now do without this department, and its support is as essential as that of any other."[3]

The department's physical limitations were the most serious problem which faced Henry Pancoast in 1902. As he later described the situation: ". . . our plant consisted of two 7-inch coils, two or three tubes, a little room on the first floor without windows, an entrance by one door too narrow for a bed to pass, dark, hot, unventilated and overcrowded, and a dark room with just enough room to permit one to turn around."[4] Despite these difficulties, however, he substantially increased the patient load, examining twice the number of patients seen in 1901 during the last six months of 1902, and expanded the department's services to include therapeutic treatment for malignant tumors in addition to the full scale diagnostic program. The therapeutic work was begun by a Dr. Rahte, a resident physician at the hospital, and was carried on during 1902 with the assistance of Mr. Bernstein, a senior in the medical school. Student interest in the project was greater than the number of patients to be treated, and two other

[21]

men were ready to help with treatments when an increase in the patient load required additional assistance.[5]

The expansion of services, as well as an increase in personnel, was clearly indicative of Dr. Pancoast's enthusiasm for his new post and of the capabilities of the department. Without evidence that added support was forthcoming from the hospital, though, he remained cautious about the rapid expansion of services like therapeutic treatments, which required considerable time, expense, and assistance, and caused great wear on the apparatus.[6]

Henry Khunrath Pancoast—Biographical Information

Henry Pancoast was born and raised in Philadelphia, the son of a physician who was also interested in light, light rays, and their relationship to medicine. He graduated from Friend's Central School in 1892, but was forced to delay his plans to study medicine due to the premature death of both his parents. Pancoast worked as a teller at the Centennial Bank, Thirty-second and Market Streets, for two years, and entered the School of Medicine at the University of Pennsylvania in 1894 without any undergraduate premedical preparation. He did very well in medical school, however, and was accorded the honor of an internship at University Hospital upon graduation.

Pancoast remained affiliated with the hospital after completing his internship, serving as an Assistant Instructor in Clinical Surgery and Assistant Demonstrator of Surgery.[7] When Dr. White approached him regarding the position in the Roentgen Ray Department he was serving as an anesthetist at the hospital and attending to a very limited outside practice, so the opportunity was both interesting and timely. He later remarked: "How easy it was in those days to become a radiologist by the shortest affirmative reply!"[8]

Growth Under Henry K. Pancoast, 1903–04

Pancoast was serious when he spoke of the need for expanded facilities and new equipment in 1902, and in the subsequent two

[22]

years the department made tremendous strides. Substantial increases in the patient load necessitated additional staff, so a nurse was borrowed from a nearby ward to prepare the women patients, part-time assistants were recruited from the second and third year medical school classes and fourth year dental school class, and another physician occasionally offered assistance.[9] In addition to his clinical duties Pancoast assumed teaching responsibilities in the medical school as the Lecturer on Skiagraphy, as well as continuing his involvement in surgical instruction.[10]

During 1903 Dr. White and the Executive Committee of the hospital's Board of Managers began to raise money to build a modern and complete X-ray facility, and by the end of the year a considerable sum had been collected.[11] Substantial income came from the Commonwealth of Pennsylvania, totaling $13,000 in 1904 and $30,000 in 1905,[12] in addition to contributions generated by private sources. These monies guaranteed the department's expansion into a first rate operation.

It was some time before the funds for the new facility were in hand and construction could actually begin, however, and in the meanwhile Dr. Pancoast was faced with severe operating constraints. The single workroom was so hot that the department was moved upstairs, to a side room off the men's surgical ward, during the summer of 1903, moved back downstairs during the winter, and back upstairs the following summer. The cramped darkroom facilities became intolerable after a period, and the hospital moved the darkroom permanently to a larger room in the basement.[13] Further improvements were made by the beginning of 1904, and although the department was not yet in its new facility, diagnosis and treatment were carried on in two separate workrooms.[14]

Gradual additions were also made to the department's stock of apparatus, and beginning in 1903 considerable sums were expended to purchase new pieces of equipment and to replace parts on old equipment so that it would be as up-to-date as possible. Three induction coils were in constant use by 1903,[15] including a new 18-inch coil, operated by a mechanical spring interrupter, which was purchased from the local Roentgen Manufacturing Company. This piece was used to make the department's first barium enema exposures, one of the most reliable abdominal examinations at that time.[16] Some other specialized equipment was also purchased, including a Sweet and Lewis tube stand and a Queen X-ray table; prior to this the department had improvised

[23]

to provide set-ups with traditional laboratory equipment.[17] By early 1904 the department had also purchased a full line of X-ray tubes, allowing considerably greater flexibility in diagnosis and therapeutic procedures.[18]

The expansion of the department's therapy work was very time consuming, not only because the treatments were often of several minutes duration (fifteen to thirty minutes at times), but also because there were no accurate ways to measure the dose or to recreate identical conditions for a later patient. Much time was spent guessing the current by the "fatness" of the spark, and these rather haphazard therapy treatments were continued for several days or weeks until a visible reaction was achieved. The intricacies of the therapy process, in addition to rather lengthy exposures for many diagnostic examinations (some spinal exposures, plus most chest, body, and hip exposures took as long as ten minutes each at this time), meant that Dr. Pancoast and his student assistants were always busy in their tiny cubical.[19]

The Fourth Annual Meeting of the American Roentgen Ray Society: Houston Hall, University of Pennsylvania, Philadelphia, December 9–10, 1903

The American Roentgen Ray Society was established in 1900 as the first national organization of physicians, physicists, and other scientists interested in working with the X-ray. Most of its members were residents of the eastern United States, and from the time of its founding it has met annually to discuss new developments and techniques and to exchange information from personal experience working with radiation.

The Fourth Annual Meeting was held in Philadelphia in December of 1903, and was hosted by the University of Pennsylvania. The Local Arrangements Committee for the meeting, Drs. Pancoast, Frazier, and Willard from University Hospital, planned an impressive and extensive two day program for the more than 300 physicians and scientists from the United States and Canada who came to the city, including the presentation of seventeen papers (each followed by a discussion lead by another specialist), a large exhibit of roentgenographic equipment (including displays by nearly all the leading manufacturers), and exhibits of prints made by a number of those in attendance. The manufacturers' displays were a particularly popular part of the program: so popular, in fact, that there was not enough room to accomodate all the companies who wished to send representatives.

The speakers came from all over the United States and covered a variety of topics, ranging from the pathological effects of X-rays on tissue to accuracy in diagnosis, from skiagraphy of the chest to danger to the operator, and from techniques for dental skiagraphs to the therapeutic effects of the X-ray. One highlight was the address by the Society's outgoing President, Arthur W. Goodspeed, entitled "The Trend of Modern Thought on the Sub-Atomic Structure of Matter" in which he outlined, from a physicist's point of view, contemporary theories about the composition of the atom.[20] Goodspeed also discussed problems arising from secondary radiation, and this concern was voiced with frequency by others in discussions of skin problems and radiation burns.[21]

Although Charles Lester Leonard was no longer affiliated with the University Hospital, his position in Philadelphia's roentgenologic community was still very important, and he presented a paper discussing his work using roentgen rays to diagnose renal calculus. He emphasized the importance of developing the diagnostic capabilities of the roentgen procedure, expressing concern that excitement generated by its newly-discovered therapeutic possibilities might minimize potential work in diagnosis, while also speaking enthusiastically about the opportunities for X-ray therapy. Recognizing Leonard as a pioneer in the field, a physician from Michigan expressed the position that: "Everyone is familiar with Dr. Leonard's work and we ought to be proud of what he has done in this line."[22]

Speaking as Skiagrapher of University Hospital, Henry Pancoast presented two distinctly different papers, one on collapsing X-ray tubes and the other on the utilization of X-rays for therapeutic purposes. The first, although brief, was interesting because it delineated a problem faced by many of his colleagues. His paper on the therapeutic use of X-rays was of major importance, however, and aroused the most interest at the convention and in the press of any presentation made at the meeting.

With the assistance of Dr. Harvey Bartle and Henry C. Welker, a second year medical student, Dr. Pancoast discussed a sample of nearly 100 patients who had been treated with X-rays for therapeutic purposes in the eighteen months that he had run the department at University Hospital. Concentrating this presentation on the treatment of tumors, Pancoast detailed both successful and unsuccessful cases, and cautioned his fellow roentgenologists against the application of X-rays as a "cure-all" for tumors, especially malignant ones. Analyzing the results of his work to date, he expressed the sentiment that ". . . up to the present time I have been very much disappointed in the results obtained from the X-ray in the treatment of cancer and sarcoma."[23]

As Dr. Pancoast pointed out, however, it was important to realize that the University Hospital X-ray laboratory was considered a "dumping ground" for all incurable cases, and a high rate of cure would be very unlikely, and could occur only if many of the department's potential patients refused treatment. In addition, most of the department's therapy patients were treated as out-patients, making only sporadic visits for treatment, and for some reason these patients seemed to arrive simultaneously, necessitating the rapid treatment of a great many persons, rather than the deliberate and individualized treatment which each patient ideally deserved.

Overall, Pancoast presented a cautious but optimistic view of the prospects for the roentgen ray therapy program: "I am not discouraged by our failures to effect cures in more cases, as I feel that we are apt to be over-enthusiastic and to expect too much of a practically new and not thoroughly understood therapeutic agent." He advised the initial removal of diseased areas by surgery wherever possible, followed by X-ray therapy, and strongly emphasized the continued necessity of surgical intervention.[24]

Dr. Pancoast's paper was interesting not only for its comments about the advances in the use of X-rays for therapeutic purposes, but also because it provided considerable insight into the situation at University Hospital in 1903. The staff, including the surgeons, was obviously willing to allow Pancoast to develop a program of X-ray therapy, but at the same time the surgical staff wanted to make certain that they were given every opportunity to remove diseased tissue surgically prior to the commencement of a radiation therapy program. DeForest Willard, a member of the Local Arrangements Committee and a surgeon at University Hospital, clearly outlined this position:

I have great confidence in the X-ray in selected cases, but I also believe that it should be employed in connection with surgical measures wherever possible. Of course, there is a large class of inoperable cases, and another class that is absolutely hopeless, and yet even in these we can remove much tissue with the knife and then fall back upon the X-ray to do the rest.[25]

The Philadelphia meeting was very successful, and attracted much notice in the local newspapers. Philadelphia roentgenologists were recognized for their many and varied contributions to this new branch of medicine, and both Charles Lester Leonard and Henry Khunrath Pancoast were elected members of the American Roentgen Ray Society at this meeting; Pancoast, in fact, had been told that he would be elected, and that he should go ahead and organize the entire program. The participation at the meeting by members of the staff of University Hospital from departments other than the X-Ray Department underscored the importance of the new specialty, as well as the status achieved by Pancoast and the department in the year-and-a-half in which he had operated it.

The New Facility: 1904–05

Especially important advances were made by the X-Ray Department in 1904, because in that year the hospital built and equipped an addition to the Agnew Pavilion, specifically for roentgenology, with the money received earlier from private sources and the Commonwealth of Pennsylvania. The expansion covered an entire floor over one of the wings of the building, facing south over the hospital grounds, and although the department began to move into the new facility in the late summer and early fall of 1904, the formal dedication was delayed until November 28th, concurrent with the Commencement Exercises for the hospital's School of Nursing.[26]

The new facility contained nine rooms, a toilet, and a sun parlor. The rooms permitted some separation of activities, and included an office and consulting room, a laboratory for pathological work (with storage space for plates), a waiting room for private patients, a waiting room for male dispensary patients, a waiting room for female dispensary patients, a store room and workshop, an X-ray room for treating gynecological patients, and a room for the major part of the therapeutic and diagnostic work. There was also a separate darkroom located, for the first time, in space adjoining the rest of the department. A glass skylight occupied two-thirds of the roof of the sun parlor, an area to be used for photography and Finsen sunlight therapy apparatus.[27]

A number of pieces of new apparatus were purchased to furnish the new facility, including a 24-inch induction coil; it was one of the largest ever made for X-ray work and was equipped with a milliammeter to ascertain the amount of current in the secondary circuit, and thereby provide some reference point for repeating procedures under similar conditions. This new coil supplemented both the 18-inch coil purchased late in 1903 and the two smaller coils, enabling the staff to transport the smaller pieces and make exposures almost anywhere inside or outside the hospital building. Two Finsen-Reyn lamps were purchased for phototherapy, in addition to a Finsen sunlight lamp and coil to provide "high frequency" treatments. Although some reservations were placed on the relative success of these Danish Finsen lights in comparison to X-ray treatment, the department made the investment to insure the absolute completeness of its new installation.[28]

Numerous purchases were also made during this year to stock the department with modern pieces of small apparatus, reflecting recent advances in X-ray technology. These included a variety of models of X-ray tubes and the most sensitive X-ray plates; various combinations were best suited for different types of exposures. The laboratory was equipped to carry out pathological and experimental work, in addition to routine urine analysis and blood examination.[29] The department was also attractively furnished, and decorated with a variety of plants and fresh flowers.

The hospital's Board of Managers was exceedingly proud of this new facility, and by the time of its completion it was ". . . believed to be the finest and most perfect of its kind in the United States."[30] Writing in the the mid-1940s Mary Virginia Stephenson, for many years Director of the hospital's School of Nursing, related that "it was stated conservatively at the time that no hospital in the country had a larger or better equipped laboratory than that of the University Hospital."[31]

It is interesting to note, however, that despite the department's enormous expansion from a single room and darkroom to a suite of nine rooms plus a sun parlor, only two rooms were designed for the utilization of X-rays and Finsen light for diagnostic and therapeutic work. The new facility enabled a great many more patients to wait for examinations and treatment, and with the

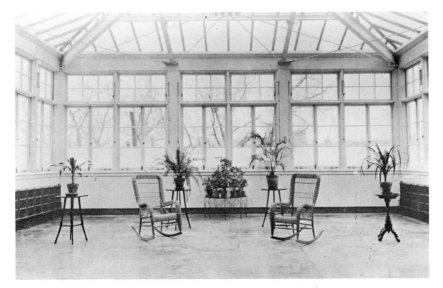

Departmental sun parlor, 1907

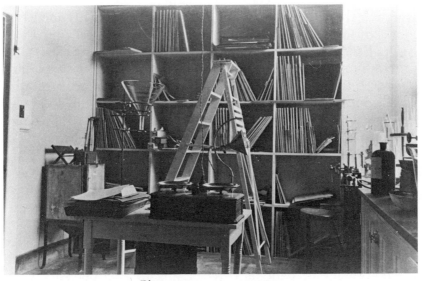

Plate storage room, 1907

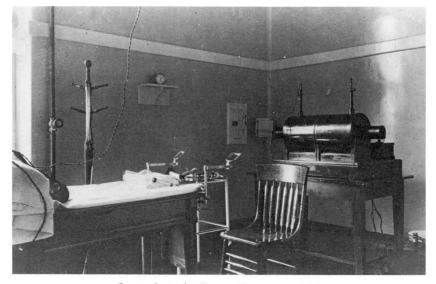

Gynecological examination room, 1907

new apparatus a great many more patients were actually seen as well, but the available working space was not actually increased very considerably.

Dr. Pancoast's report for the year ending August 31, 1905 provides some particularly interesting insights into the expanded operation and the new facility, approximately nine months after the beginning of routine activity. The space was utilized at all times, and the laboratory and workrooms enabled the application of surgical dressings in the laboratory instead of in the wards or surgical dispensary, as well as the performance of necessary minor surgical operations in the department itself. There was a marked increase in the amount of diagnostic X-ray work performed during the year, and an even greater increase in the application of X-ray and other treatments for therapy. X-rays, radium, Finsen light, and high frequency (Finsen sunlight) therapy were all used in treatment, and there was an encouraging increase in the percentage of patients cured, rising to 23.5 percent of the cases treated.[32] This figure is especially impressive in view of the 10 percent cure rate quoted by Dr. Pancoast in his 1903 observations on the success of X-rays as therapeutic agents.

The increase in the patient load undoubtedly necessitated staff increases, and it seems very likely that students from the University's medical and dental schools continued to participate in the department's work, both in treatment and research projects. The expansion did require the addition of a full-time nurse to attend to the women patients, and a second or third year student nurse was assigned this responsibility.[33]

The extension of University Hospital's roentgenology program was further reflected in the work being done independently by Dr. Louis Duhring in the Dispensary for Skin Diseases. Dr. Pancoast had made it clear from the beginning that he felt skin diseases were the responsibility of the dermatologists, since they had the necessary expertise in this field, and early in 1904 Dr. Duhring purchased a roentgen ray plant, including an 18-inch coil, for his own work. The expansion of Dr. Pancoast's program is particularly remarkable, therefore, since he was not seeing patients with skin diseases or counting them among his ever increasing patient load.

Dr. Pancoast's enthusiasm for the potential of X-rays and related procedures for both diagnostic and therapeutic purposes did not blind him to the very present dangers from overexposure to the rays, however. The painful and tragic experience of his predecessor, in addition to those of a number of Philadelphia roentgenologists, was an ever present caution, and he was mindful to purchase lead foil and other protective devices to shield both operator and patient from secondary radiation and prolonged exposure to the still-mysterious X-rays.

The Establishment of the Philadelphia Roentgen Ray Society—1905

Philadelphia was the home of a number of pioneers in the field of roentgenology, and in February, 1905, Charles Lester Leonard invited a dozen of these men to his private office to organize a local society for the ". . . study of the roentgen rays and the formation of friendly intercourse." The group included the physicians responsible for roentgenology departments in Philadelphia hospitals, plus specialists in other medical fields and scientists and engineers who were in some way involved in the development of this new specialty. A number of corresponding members, individuals prominent in roentgenology in other cities, were also elected, and some were occasionally able to attend meetings.

From its beginning the Society was interested in protection for the X-ray operator, as well as in new developments in the field. A number of early discussions concentrated on protection, the introduction of new devices to provide safer working conditions, and the treatment of X-ray dermatitis. Members also brought plates from unusual or difficult cases to the meetings, and informal discussions evolved, providing an early precedent for the city-wide film reading sessions which were later organized at University Hospital and at Society meetings.

Through the enthusiastic efforts of Drs. Leonard, Pancoast, and others, the Society organized symposia on topics of interest and importance to the growing number of roentgenologists in the Philadelphia area, in addition to providing input at national meetings. Throughout its history the roentgenologists from University Hospital have actively supported the programs of the Philadelphia Roentgen Ray Society and played an important role in its expansion and growth.[34]

Continued Expansion of Services: 1905–11

The X-Ray Department firmly established its permanency and professionalism with the move to its new facility in 1904, but a fire in the University's power house in 1905 caused many frustrations for Dr. Pancoast and his staff. The hospital turned to the city for temporary electrical current, but the alternating current thus supplied was not compatible with the department's apparatus and it was necessary to string wires from Philadelphia General Hospital to University Hospital for four months during the winter of 1905–06 to supply the X-Ray Department with direct current. The arrangement proved very inconvenient at times, because the voltage was likely to drop considerably in the course of a roentgenographic exposure, but after a while the staff learned to compensate and minimize the difficulty.[35]

During these years the department experienced an overwhelming increase in its patient load in response to both diagnostic and therapeutic innovations. Dr. Pancoast's work with salts of bismuth in 1906 enabled diagnosis of obscure conditions of the gastrointestinal tract, and for the first time analysis of many of these deep areas of the body was possible.[36] The Finsen light treatment proved rather unsuccessful for therapeutic purposes, but the department relied on the high frequency treatment with increasing regularity during this period. In addition, more and more X-ray treatments were administered each year.

The fluoroscope was introduced into the department's diagnostic procedure on a large scale for the first time in 1906, but concern for the operator minimized the utilization of this equipment during this period. In addition to difficulties suffered by Philadelphia roentgenologists, the department's first permanent nurse had received a partial epilation due to overexposure. She returned a few years later to be treated for leukemia, from which she died shortly thereafter. Dr. Pancoast was continually concerned about safety and protection, however, and it was not until 1913, when improvements in design minimized the danger to the operator, that fluoroscopes were used extensively.

Early in this period the department began to use filters in addition to taking the precaution, when possible, of surrounding the tube with a box covered with lead paint. Lead foil was frequently employed for filters, as was leather soaked in water to resemble skin. The leather proved rather unsuccessful, and was soon replaced by metal and wood.[37]

The department's equipment was kept up-to-date, and Dr. Pancoast had at his disposal a variety of tubes and other pieces of apparatus with which to perform many different procedures. The department's new 24-inch coil was used for both therapeutic and diagnostic work, but with different interrupters to provide different kinds and amounts of current. A mechanical spring interrupter was used for therapy because it provided minimum secondary current and softer, more absorbent rays, while an electrolytic interrupter was used for diagnosis because it produced harder rays.

Dr. Pancoast used many different brands of gas tubes, trying new designs as they were introduced on the market, and found that a good gas tube could be used to make several hundred exposures, barring an accident. The vacuum within individual tubes changed frequently, however, even though the self-regulating tube was used extensively. Sometimes the vacuum dropped so much after three or four minutes of operation that it was necessary to use three or four different tubes to complete a lengthy therapy treatment. Success varied more with individual tubes than individual manufacturers, and Dr. Pancoast and his assistants each developed pet tubes which they would use again and again.[38]

A particularly important development in X-ray equipment, the Snook transformer, simplified the department's work immeasurably during this period. H. Clyde Snook, a Philadelphia engineer and founding member of the Philadelphia Roentgen Ray Society, had been involved for some time in the development of a new and improved apparatus for X-ray production. He designed the milliammeter for the department's 24-inch induction coil, built an improved induction coil, and in 1908, after experimentation in the University's Department of Physics, provided the department with its first transformer. The most important advantage of this new apparatus was the elimination of the need for an interrupter to change the available direct into alternating potential for the X-ray equipment. This meant that the department could use powerful alternating current, available from the University's power plant or directly from the city, and transform it into the voltage required for X-ray production.

The Snook transformer made the process of diagnostic examination both easier and more effective, and in 1908 and 1909 the department began extensive stomach roentgenology in earnest. A device built in the department's workshop enabled the exposure of plates in an erect position, thereby minimizing the difficulty of examining this portion of the anatomy. In 1909 the department also added an "Improved Sweet Localizer," a piece of apparatus used primarily to locate foreign bodies in the eyes, thus reinforcing cooperative activities with other departments in the hospital. Dr. deSchweinitz, the chief ophthalmologist, was particularly interested in this apparatus, and he raised most of the money for its purchase.[39]

Henry Pancoast encouraged students to assist him in the X-ray laboratory soon after he became hospital skiagrapher in 1902, and over the years students had participated in a variety of projects, particularly ones related to studies of the therapuetic capabilities of the X-ray. After the opening of the large facility, participation gradually increased, and by 1909 the department's status was such that the *Annual Report of the Board of Managers* listed additional personnel, including a physician serving as Assistant in the X-Ray Department, along with the rest of the hospital's medical staff.[40] This recognition of importance was relayed in other publications as well, including the 1910 issue of the Medical School

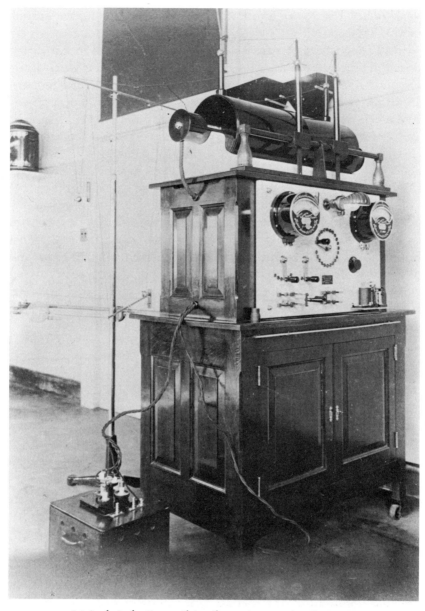

24-inch induction coil in the main examination room,
1907

yearbook: "The X-ray Laboratory has become a valuable branch of the Hospital."[41]

Dr. Pancoast and his associates carried out a great many varied research projects, most with direct application to their work at the hospital, in addition to their routine clinical and teaching responsibilities. Diagnostic work during this period included cooperative work with Charles Frazier, a neurosurgeon, on the diagnosis and examination of brain lesions, and considerable work on the gastrointestinal tract. Pancoast's development of the bismuth shadow, and later work to develop a similar substance without the allergic properties of bismuth, were particularly important.

During this period Dr. Pancoast also began an especially important series of research projects on the therapeutic possibilities of the X-ray, expanding the work he had begun in 1903. Most important was the beginning of the treatment of leukemia and other diseases of the blood-producing organs, a venture involving close cooperation with the hospital's Department of Medicine. He also became interested in the chest at this time, and expended much energy in the treatment of tuberculosis with X-rays.

Overall, the years following the move into the new installation served firmly to establish the department as an indispensable professional service to University Hospital. The continuous increases in staff and the scope of services offered were the beginning of a process which still continues.

The Nation's First Professor of Roentgenology—1911

Henry K. Pancoast was appointed Lecturer on Skiagraphy for the 1903–04 academic year, and held that position until the spring of 1911 when the University's Trustees received the somewhat unusual nomination of Pancoast as a full professor in the School of Medicine, bypassing the usual intermediate ranks. His election as a Professor, recommended at the March Trustees' meeting, was delayed a month until a legal quorum was present, and on April 4, 1911 "a ballot was so cast and Dr. H. K. Pancoast duly elected Professor of Roentgenology."[42]

Controversy has arisen over whether or not Henry Pancoast was the first physician to achieve the rank of full professor in the relatively new field of roentgenology, and a number of authors have named George E. Pfahler, another Philadelphian, as the first man to receive this honor. A close look at the details of Pfahler's particular situation, however, refutes any possible claim he might have to the first professorship.

During the years just prior to 1911 George E. Pfahler was working and teaching at the Medico-Chirurgical College, located at Seventeenth and Cherry Streets in Philadelphia. In recognition of his excellent work at this institution, and the service he was rendering both the College and the Hospital, he was elected to fill a newly-created position of Clinical Professor of Roentgenology in December, 1909. At the meeting of the Medico-Chi Trustees in October, 1912, it was evident, however, that Dr. Pfahler was displeased with this position because it did not include all the normal privileges associated with the rank of Professor, and he indicated that he was likely to leave the institution if changes were not forthcoming. The situation was resolved at the December, 1912 meeting, when ". . . Doctor Pfahler was elected Professor of Roentgenology, said election to include a chair in the voting Faculty." His election to a full professorship came twenty months after that of Henry Pancoast, making Pfahler the second Professor of Roentgenology in the city and nation.[43]

The creation of a Professorship in Roentgenology for Henry Pancoast in 1911 was indicative of the prestige which he and his department had achieved in both the hospital and School of Medicine. The new appointment also changed his hospital title, and thereafter he was the Roentgenologist.[44] His promotion occasioned the first roentgenology course description in the *University Catalog,* and the program for the 1911–12 academic year was delineated as:

ROENTGENOLOGY. Professor Pancoast.—A series of lectures and demonstrations covering the diagnostic and therapeutic application of X-rays, and the interpretation of radiograms.[45]

Equally rewarding, perhaps, was Pancoast's acceptance by the medical students as a full-fledged member of the teaching faculty. His tribute in the 1911 yearbook seems most clearly to reflect this position:

Our Pancoast thinks everyone crazy
Who works without skiagrams hazy,
    In fact you would laugh

[37]

To hear the whole staff
Rave on as if they were X-rasy.[46]

Growth and National Recognition Before World War I

The X-Ray Department's reputation extended far beyond the University, and within a short period of time Henry K. Pancoast was a leader of both the Philadelphia and national roentgenological communities. He was an active participant in the Philadelphia Post-Graduate School of Roentgenology, organized by the Philadelphia Roentgen Ray Society in 1913 to provide graduate training to interested physicians, and he always encouraged interested persons to visit the department at University Hospital.[47] After Charles Lester Leonard's death in 1913, the Philadelphia Society which he had established was reorganized, and Pancoast was elected Vice President that year and President two years later.[48]

Pancoast's reputation had spread far beyond the city, and following the 1903 meeting of the American Roentgen Ray Society in Philadelphia people remained interested in this young physician. He was elected Secretary of that Society in 1911, and elected President the following year, thus involving him in considerable outside activity in addition to his continually expanding responsibilities at University Hospital. Pancoast's accomplishments, capability, and cordiality continued to impress his colleagues, and he was elected a charter member of the American Radium Society when it was established in 1916, its Secretary in 1917, and its President two years later.[49]

Through their joint activities in Philadelphia roentgenology, Pancoast and Leonard remained close friends, particularly since they shared an interest in the diagnostic examination of the gastrointestinal tract. Leonard was asked to give a paper on the history of gastrointestinal examinations at the Radiology Section of the International Congress in London in 1913. He was too ill to complete the work so he called on Pancoast, and the younger man abstracted the topic and presented it to the gathering for Leonard. Such a request indicates the extent of their friendship, as well as Leonard's confidence in Pancoast's abilities.

The most exciting development in the department during the years before the war was the introduction of an extensive program of radium therapy. Radium had been used briefly by Dr. Pancoast in 1905,[50] but the lack of sufficient financial resources had prevented the implementation of a full scale program at that time. In 1914 George H. McFadden, a member of the hospital's Board of Managers, gave money to purchase 100 milligrams of radium.[51] The following year Dr. Charles H. Frazier arranged for an additional 125 milligrams, provided by another generous donor, to be transferred to Dr. Pancoast for safekeeping and use in treatment.[52] Pancoast was enthusiastic about the possibilities for therapeutic advances using radium, but unfamiliar with the techniques of its application, so shortly after the department's acquisition he spent a day in New York for instruction and advice in the proper application of radium for treatment with Dr. Robert Abbe, a physician whose work with radium had brought him national prominence.[53]

Dr. Pancoast used radium to treat a variety of symptoms and diseases, including inoperable carcinoma, brain tumors, uterine hemorrhaging, warts, and moles.[54] A Caldwell cavity tube was used to treat tumors in inaccessible locations such as the mouth, rectum, and uterus.[55] Radium treatment of gynecological cases was so successful that Dr. Pancoast, realizing his limitations in this specialty, encouraged Dr. John G. Clark to procure his own radium supply,[56] and by 1917 Clark was treating these cases himself.[57]

New equipment was purchased as the need arose and the patient load increased, and beginning in 1913 the fluoroscope was used extensively. Improvements in this apparatus had now alleviated earlier fears, and it was used on hundreds of patients. Coolidge tubes were also introduced in 1913, eventually replacing gas tubes and promoting much greater efficiency in the department's work. Intensifying screens, purchased from a German firm at the beginning of the decade and from an American firm just prior to and during the war, substantially improved the quality of the exposures.[58]

By 1916 the department was very cramped in its quarters in the Agnew Wing, and plans were begun to move it to space in the new surgical building, a tribute to J. William White, which was then under construction. This building had been started several years before but never completed, and in 1916 a special fund was initiated to raise money so that a portion of the first floor of the building could be finished immediately for use by the X-Ray Department. Space in the Agnew Wing office was at such a premium, in fact, that no increases in diagnostic work were possible. All unnecessary work was reduced to a minimum, and all work from the Dental Department was transferred to the Dental School, thereby slightly decreasing the overall patient load.[59]

Henry Pancoast's interest in a variety of diagnostic and therapeutic research projects continued during this time, and he expanded the program, begun earlier with the assistance of Dr. Alfred Stengel, of treating bone marrow as the primary site of leukemia. Dr. Pancoast's earlier interest in research on the chest, and the analysis of roentgenographic examinations of tuberculosis patients, expanded in 1915 to include the study of workers in environments where organic dusts were produced and settled in the lungs. This project was an ongoing one and was enthusiastically expanded by his associates in subsequent years.[60]

The real urgency requiring the move of the X-Ray Department to new quarters was gradually realized by the hospital's Board of Managers, and during 1917 they raised nearly $25,000 for the completion of the available space in the White Building. The situation was particularly critical since the Agnew Wing office had only enough space to handle one treatment case at a time, and since most patients made between one and ten visits in the course of the year, often for rather lengthy periods of time, there were serious backlogs in the therapy program. The construction of the new facility was well underway during the summer of 1917, and the project's necessity was publicly affirmed by the Board of Managers: ". . . it will provide the Hospital with adequate facilities for the housing and equipment of the X-ray Department, the use of which has become of such increasing importance in all branches of the Hospital's work."[61]

The department's growth during this period also extended to the expansion of graduate medical education, since the 1916 merger of the Medico-Chirurgical College with the University's School of Medicine formed the beginning of the Graduate School of Medicine of the University of Pennsylvania. The opportunities for graduate education in roentgenology, organized as a formal curriculum, promised expansion of the earlier efforts of the Philadelphia Roentgen Ray Society, and offered the initiation of new projects at University Hospital to support this growing program.

Departmental Operations During the War Years

Planning for the department's cooperative efforts in graduate education in roentgenology continued during the war years, although the formal classes in the Graduate School of Medicine did not begin until 1919. The Philadelphia Polyclinic Hospital and College merged with the University's School of Medicine in 1917, and the faculty of the Polyclinic became the nucleus of the graduate school's clinical staff. Dr. Pancoast and one of the Assistant Roentgenologists on his staff, as well as staff and faculty from the other institutions, presented formal lectures from the outset of the program.[62] Unlike the organization at University Hospital and the University's School of Medicine, however, roentgenology was recognized as a separate discipline in the graduate school structure, and a Department of Radiology, charged with developing its own curriculum, was established under Dr. George E. Pfahler.[63]

Soon after the beginning of United States involvement in the First World War, Dr. Pancoast and his staff became involved in a program to educate medical officers in the specifics of roentgenologic technique, adding another responsibility to their already overtaxed schedules. Some portions of the instruction were routine and taught in conjunction with the undergraduate medical school courses, but additional instruction placed special emphasis on the various methods of foreign body localization. The use of the roentgenoscope was encouraged, as was the value and necessity of methods of localization which were faster, though less safe, than those in use in regular civilian practice. Most of Dr. Pancoast's students were surgeons, and it was his responsibility to teach them all the available methods and to encourage them to use their own judgment to determine which would be the most speedy, accurate, and comfortable for a particular patient.[64]

The hospital records indicate that there were two Assistant Roentgenologists associated with the department during these years, but since these physicians also spent time at other hospitals, Dr. Pancoast still carried most of the departmental workload. Visiting graduate students, from other parts of the nation or abroad, often spent two or three weeks in the department, but they were here for training and were not part of the productive staff.[65]

In 1918 University Hospital offered the customary internships to the students graduating at the very top of the class from the University's School of Medicine. A great many of these young men enlisted in the service, however, and the hospital soon found itself without an adequate supply of interns to function effectively. The President of the University persuaded the Navy to send a number of the doctors working at the Philadelphia Naval Yard, who had originally planned to do internships, back to University Hospital. Among the group was Eugene Percival Pendergrass, who was assigned to assist Dr. Pancoast in the Department of Roentgenology.

Dr. Pendergrass's tour of duty with the Navy was begun as an intern at University Hospital, and after a while he persuaded Dr. Pancoast that he, too, should enlist. Dr. Pancoast did join the Navy, and soon became an important consultant to the Philadelphia Naval Hospital and other Navy medical installations.[66] His work required a fair amount of travel, which resulted in his absence from the hospital. During this time Dr. Pendergrass was of great assistance in coordinating the move of the department from its quarters in the Agnew Wing to the new installation on the first floor of the J. William White Surgical Pavilion.[67]

While at University Hospital Dr. Pendergrass was asked to undertake a roentgenologic study of a number of British seamen who arrived in Philadelphia very ill, and who, it was later discovered, brought the influenza virus to the city that caused the 1918 epidemic. Dr. Pendergrass's assignment to work with Dr. Pancoast at University Hospital was cut short because the Navy needed his expertise to diagnose sailors suffering from influenza, but he later returned to the hospital and completed the full rotation of his internship.

During these years all actual X-ray examinations were made by physicians in the department, with nurses assisting as technicians. Dr. Pancoast was very particular about his personnel requirements for staff members: except for a few special cases all of the technicians were registered nurses. The calibre of his staff and his concern for protection for both operator and patient were but two indications of Dr. Pancoast's demand for excellence and the very best in roentgenologic procedures. His reputation was international by this time, and physicians from all over the world would visit him when they were in the United States.[68]

Dr. Pancoast was able successfully to keep the hospital's X-ray plant modern and up-to-date, although during these years batteries connected by bare wires were still used to make exposures outside the hospital. The same unreliable gas tubes were still used, and each physician continued to reserve a pet tube—or tubes—for his own use.[69] Therapy work was not limited to the Department of Roentgenology. In addition to Dr. Clark's work in the Department of Gynecology, Dr. Pancoast's first memory of losing a tube of radium involved its loan to a laryngologist to treat a growth on the nose.[70]

The therapy cases in the Department of Roentgenology were just about equally divided between treatment of malignant disease and treatment of inflammatory conditions at this time. Gas gangrene was treated primarily with X-rays, as were leukemia, Hodgkin's Disease, skin cancer, and recurrent breast cancer. Radium was used to treat cancer of the cervix. The department experienced some success in controlling brain tumors, and treatment of tuberculosis of the lymph nodes was very common. In general, the roentgenologist was usually consulted as a last resort when there was no other alternative for patient treatment. The more experience a roentgenologist gained treating a variety of symptoms and diseases, the safer he was considered to supervise a course of treatment.[71]

Despite the move to the White Pavilion, Dr. Pancoast's sporadic absence for consulting work for the Navy and the absence of several members of the staff due to long term military obligations, the department continued to increase its patient load and expand its services to the hospital community during the war years. Eugene P. Pendergrass's brief assignment to the department in 1918 convinced him to return to work with Dr. Pancoast after completing his internship at the hospital. His participation would shape much of the department's future.

Eugene Percival Pendergrass— Early Biographical Information

Eugene Percival Pendergrass was raised in South Carolina, the son of a merchant. He wanted very much to go to college, although difficulties in the cotton market prevented his father from sending him, but a kind gentleman agreed to loan Eugene Pendergrass the necessary funds, and in the fall of 1912 he began studying at Wofford College in Spartansburg, South Carolina.

Pendergrass spent his summers grading cotton and working in laundries, and after two years of college decided to apply to medical school rather than complete his undergraduate degree at Wofford. He was accepted into the two year medical program at the University of North Carolina and entered classes there in the fall of 1914. The North Carolina program did not offer a Doctor of Medicine degree, however, so in the fall of 1916 he changed institutions once again and was accepted as a member of the third year class in the School of Medicine at the University of Pennsylvania. He graduated among the top twenty-five students in his class in 1918, and was offered an internship at University Hospital which he accepted.

Pendergrass was in the Army in 1918 when the United States became involved in the war. He feared he would never leave Philadelphia if he remained in the Army, however, so he took the examination for the Navy, passed it, and was immediately sent to the Naval Hospital on Greys Ferry Road. Unfortunately for him, though, he was one of the interns sent back to University Hospital when their staffing shortage became critical. He was assigned to the Department of Roentgenology, and his initial reaction was one of displeasure and frustration: "I thought I had spent four years in medicine and two years in college, and to end up taking pictures just didn't appeal to me very much."[72] He quickly discovered just how lucky he was to be working with Dr. Pancoast in roentgenology, however, and soon his fellow interns were all quite jealous.

Due to staffing shortages caused by the war, he remained in the department for several months longer than he might have under a regular internship rotation and might have remained even longer had the city not been hit by the influenza epidemic. After working with Dr. Pancoast on the carriers of the virus, he was reassigned to the Naval Hospital to care for the marine and naval personnel who had also contracted the disease. When the epidemic became more severe, he was put in charge of an emergency hospital set up at the Medico-Chirurgical College Hospital at Seventeenth and Cherry Streets, serving as officer of the day there. He eventually contracted influenza himself, and was confined to the Naval Hospital until he recuperated.

Following his illness Pendergrass was sent to sea, and he served on four or five Atlantic crossings on a transport ship. He was offered the opportunity to study abroad after his tour of duty with the Navy was completed, but had already returned to the

United States when the delayed offer reached him. Instead he returned to University Hospital to complete his internship, and spent time rotating through a number of departments in the institution. After his training he decided he would like to specialize in roentgenology. He had an offer to return to his home town, as well as one to study at the Medical College of Virginia. However, Dr. Pancoast offered him the opportunity to remain at University Hospital and study with him. Dr. Pendergrass chose to remain in Philadelphia.

Eugene Pendergrass formally joined the staff of the Department of Roentgenology in 1920, after completing his internship, but it was a year or two before he was licensed to practice medicine in the Commonwealth of Pennsylvania. The difficulty arose over a 1914 Pennsylvania law requiring that medical students complete all their premedical training before entering medical school, and the fact that Pendergrass had taken a premedical botany course during his first year in medical school. In order to resolve the situation a new law had to be passed, outlining exceptions to the earlier one.[73]

Growth and Expansion During the 1920s

During the early 1920s there was a steady increase in the amount of therapeutic and diagnostic work carried on by the department, but no increase in the number of physicians on the staff. From 1923 until 1928 Eugene Pendergrass, serving as Assistant Roentgenologist and Assistant Director of the Clinic, was the only staff physician working with Dr. Pancoast. Interns seem to have begun rotating through the department again in 1924; they were responsible for providing twenty-four–hour emergency roentgenologic service, but during these years Dr. Pendergrass came in to take every night call, with the intern serving as his technician.[74]

The early 1920s showed an enormous growth in the number of patients treated in the department, as well as additions in space and apparatus for therapy. In 1922 a one-story building was erected south of the surgical building to house the orthopedic gymnasium while the space formerly occupied by the gymnasium, on the south side of the main corridor across the hall from the X-ray department, was given to the department to permit expansion of the therapy facilities.[75] The space was partitioned into a number of rooms, and one of the old therapy machines was remodeled and installed there. In 1923 Mr. and Mrs. Caleb F. Fox gave the department a high-voltage, deep therapy apparatus, that was also installed in the new therapy facility. Other available space was remodeled into examination and treatment space for patients receiving radium therapy, thus enabling the entire therapy program to operate in a single area. The department, always well known for its diagnostic work, could now be equally proud of its therapy facilities: "The added room and the new high-voltage deep therapy X-Ray equipment make it possible to handle all varieties of cases in which radiation treatment is indicated and have placed this Hospital in the front ranks of those in this counry for the administration of X-Ray and radium treatment."[76]

Radium played an important part in the department's therapy program, and gifts of radium or money with which to purchase radium were always necessary and welcomed. Professor R. A. F. Penrose, Jr., who had given radium to the hospital in 1918, donated $1,000 in 1924 to the Radium Fund,[77] and the following year George H. McFadden, a member of the Board of Managers who had been treated in the department, raised $3,000, enabling him to present 50 milligrams of radium to the department in the form of needles.[78] Radium in this form was first used in the department in 1921, after Dr. Pancoast requested permission from the Board of Managers to have some of the radium supply on hand put into needles. These were inserted into a growth, particularly to treat an area like the tongue.[79] When Dr. John G. Clark died in 1927, Dr. Pancoast was given responsibility for the 100 milligrams of radium which Dr. Clark had used to treat gynecological patients.[80]

The department made a major technical change about 1923, changing from single-coated glass plates to single-coated and double-coated X-ray film. The plates produced beautifully clear X-ray exposures, because there was emulsion on only one side of the glass, but they were cumbersome to handle, and since only one intensifying screen could be used the patient had to be exposed to the X-rays for a considerable period of time. The double emulsion film enabled the utilization of two intensifying screens, considerably decreasing the length of exposure, although the small added depth of the second emulsion had a tendency to produce a double image. This film not only decreased the exposure time, thereby minimizing danger for the operator and patient, but it also eliminated a great deal of motion blurring since it was easier for the patient to hold his breath. The decreased period of exposure also made it much easier to examine children.[81]

The expansion of the department's therapy program in the early 1920s was paralleled by expansion and improvements in the diagnostic program during the second half of the 1920s. The vastly increased patient load and continual utilization of equipment necessitated substantial renovations. In 1926 the hospital undertook such a program. Approximately $10,000 was spent to remodel and design the rooms, and new equipment was purchased to enable two independent diagnostic groups to work simultaneously. More than half of the money, some $7,000, was appropriated by the Board of Managers, and the balance was contributed from other sources. These improvements kept the diagnostic division apace with the impressive additions to the therapy program, and helped to maintain the high calibre of the department's operation.[82]

Expansion of the diagnostic program continued in 1927 with research on technique and equipment to more capably assist the Bronchoscopic Clinic. Many patients visiting this clinic arrived as emergency cases, and the recent modifications to the X-ray department and purchase of new equipment enabled it immediately to care for these patients when they reached the hospital. Equipment was also modified to enable the utilization of fluoroscopic procedures to extract foreign bodies from the esophagus and air passages, providing a technique for which patients were formerly sent to other institutions.[83]

By 1928 the department had developed along two lines: two general examination units, with rooms, apparatus and staff, used continually for routine diagnostic work; and separate arrangements for special, time-consuming diagnostic procedures. This separation of diagnostic activities enabled the department to function as effectively as possible in its limited space, and minimized delays in service to other departments in the hospital. The entire institution had grown to rely so heavily on the X-ray department's work that delays in diagnosis often increased the period of hospitalization of patients, at a considerable expense to the hospital. The new system of operation was designed to prevent this from happening.[84] There were further physical renovations in the department in 1929 that facilitated procedures and increased protection for the staff. A considerable amount of new equipment was also added, enabling the department to keep abreast of new technological developments.[85]

The department showed considerable growth during the decade of the 1920s: in the expansion of services and space, in the installation of up-to-date equipment, and in the gradual addition of staff at all levels. The first residents began working in the department in 1928,[86] representing a commitment to an extensive graduate training program by the department's staff. By the end of the decade there was an additional staff physician, plus one or more resident physicians, but the increase in the patient load and in the scope of the department's operation meant that the two senior staff men were incredibly busy, particularly since the residents rotated throughout the hospital during a portion of their training and were then not available as assistants. The department's spirited response to its growth and expansion during the 1920s laid a strong foundation for the following years, however, and placed the department in the forefront of the field of roentgenology.

The Moore School X-Ray Laboratory

Research using roentgenology was being pursued elsewhere in the University as well, and in 1923 F. Maurice McPhedran, M.D., an affiliate of the Henry Phipps Institute at the University, approached Harold Pender, Ph.D., Dean of the Moore School of Electrical Engineering, for assistance with his X-ray apparatus. Dr. McPhedran was a specialist on tuberculosis, but was having difficulty producing the quality X-ray films he wanted and needed for his work. He was hopeful that one of the electrical engineers at the Moore School might be able to assist him. Charles Weyl, an Instructor at the Moore School, expressed an interest in the project, and in 1924 the two men began work on a pulse relay device which caused exposure of the X-ray at a predetermined phase in the cardiac cycle.

Charles Weyl served as Director of the Moore School X-Ray Laboratory, which was formally established in Room 210 of the Moore School building and was equipped to test X-ray equipment and to conduct experiments on roentgenographic procedures. McPhedran and Weyl began studies of apparatus and techniques for chest roentgenography in 1924. This work was eventually supported by the National Tuberculosis Association, through its Medical Research Committee, and by a number of life insurance companies which were concerned about their losses from tuberculosis.

The funding from the National Tuberculosis Association began in 1929 and supported a program with three specific goals: the determination of the most effective X-ray equipment on the market and the analysis of ways to improve the apparatus; the analysis of chest roentgenography in tuberculosis sanatoria and the delineation of the best techniques to produce the optimum exposure possible in chest roentgenography; and the education of physicians in the peculiarities of chest roentgenography and in the latest developments in improved technique. The program was funded by the National Tuberculosis Association until the mid-1940s and produced many important developments in the field of chest roentgenography.

The staff of the Moore School Laboratory included S. Reid Warren, Jr., Dallett B. O'Neill and, for brief periods of time, C. Justus Garrahan and Ralph M. Showers. They were able to persuade three manufacturers of X-ray equipment to lend them apparatus to make exposures under controlled conditions in the laboratory. The results of their analyses were reported to the manufacturers as well as referred to in subsequent publications. The results of their research on various types of apparatus also proved useful in the second phase of their research for the National Tuberculosis Association, a series of site analyses of apparatus and techniques for chest roentgenography in tuberculosis sanatoria.

From 1933 until 1938, consultation visits were made to about two hundred sanatoria and hospitals in the United States and eastern Canada. Dr. Warren, usually with the help of an assistant, analyzed apparatus and procedures in each institution and made recommendations for changes which would produce an improved roentgenographic product. In addition, the laboratory's staff was involved in a considerable amount of consultation work and prepared specifications for new equipment purchases for various institutions. These specifications were unique, because they described the results that should be achieved by a specific piece of equipment, rather than a description of design and dimensions.

The third goal of the program, the dissemination of information to physicians concerning advances and improvements in the roentgenographic process, was carried out through a series of published papers and through exhibits at national meetings of the National Tuberculosis Association, the American Medical Association, the Radiological Society of North America, and the American Roentgen Ray Society.

By 1943 it became obvious that the goals of the work for the National Tuberculosis Association were nearly achieved, and that work was terminated in 1945 when the grant from the Association was expended. The faculty of the Moore School continued to work cooperatively with a number of medical departments at the University, including the Department of Roentgenology, but the Moore School's own laboratory completed its independent work in chest roentgenology with the completion of work for the National Tuberculosis Association. For a period of twenty years, however, this laboratory made extremely valuable contributions to the improvement and development of techniques and apparatus in chest roentgenography.[87]

National Participation and Awards

The high national regard held for University Hospital's Department of Roentgenology and its staff was evident in the honors achieved by members outside the University community and by the participation of these physicians in a number of national projects.

Henry Pancoast, long interested in chest roentgenology and the study of various lung diseases, was appointed chairman of a committee from the American Roentgen Ray Society which studied the appearance of the healthy chest in children and adults for the National Tuberculosis Association. His election as chairman from 1920 until 1926 was only one indication of his prominence, particularly in this branch of roentgenology.[88]

In 1928 Henry Pancoast served as chairman of the committee from the American Roentgen Ray Society charged with recommending an official nomenclature for the specialty. The American Medical Association appointed a committee composed of members of the Radiological Section and other allied radiological organizations at their annual meeting that year to consider the same questions. The report submitted by Pancoast on behalf of the American Roentgen Ray Society was adopted by the Section on Radiology of the American Medical Association, even prior to its adoption by the American Roentgen Ray Society.[89]

The expansion of the department's staff to include residents permitted the staff some free time to pursue areas of special interest in individual and joint research projects. Physicians in the department received a great many awards for research projects, papers, and exhibits at various meetings of radiological and medical societies in the late 1920s and early 1930s, for projects covering a variety of fields of interest.[90]

The greatest recognition of Dr. Pancoast's contributions to the science of roentgenology and of his accomplishments at University Hospital was his election as President of the First American Congress of Radiology in 1933.

Roentgenographic Assistance at Nearby Hospitals

In addition to expanded services and facilities at University Hospital and considerable participation in activities on the national level, the Department of Roentgenology also provided advice and assistance for roentgenographic operations at nearby hospitals.

In the late 1920s Henry Pancoast was closely involved with the establishment, in the northeastern section of the city, of Jeanes Hospital, a hospital and rest home for ailing members of the Society of Friends. Serving as consultant, he was to set up the X-Ray Department, and he asked Eugene Pendergrass to design this installation and choose a physician to run the department, which he did. The staff at University Hospital remained in close touch even after the department at Jeanes began to function, although they had no direct responsibilities there. In later years residents from University Hospital served rotations in this department, giving them an opportunity to work in an entirely different hospital setting from that at the University.

The staff at University Hospital became directly involved in the roentgenographic operation at Chestnut Hill Hospital in the late 1920s when the roentgenologist there died suddenly. Dr. Pancoast agreed to take over the operation of that department, and Dr. Pendergrass was assigned to spend several hours there each day. Severe time constraints hindered this operation somewhat, since Pendergrass routinely made rounds to speak to each patient prior to his examination, and thus many nonemergency examinations were postponed until the morning following the consultation. The patient load was sufficiently large that additional assistance was soon needed, and beginning in 1930 residents from the department at University Hospital spent time at Chestnut Hill Hospital, working with Dr. Pendergrass.

Working at Jeanes and Chestnut Hill Hospitals enabled the staff and residents from University Hospital to spend time in community hospital settings and to gain exposure to the unique aspects of this kind of roentgenographic operation. It was particularly valuable for physicians still in training, because it provided experience in the kind of environment in which many would later find themselves working permanently.[91]

New Approaches to Radiology in the Early 1930s

The decade of the 1930s had an auspicious beginning when the Department of Roentgenology at University Hospital and in the School of Medicine officially became the Department of Radiology and the staff titles were changed accordingly.[92] This followed Dr. Pancoast's term of service as chairman of the American Roentgen Ray Society's committee on nomenclature, and represented a change of mental attitude as well as semantics.

By this time radiology was beginning to be accepted as a precise, scientific field of medicine, much as surgery, and was no longer regarded unilaterally as "picture-taking" or only as a final alternative for patients whose diseases and conditions were incurable. The acceptance of radiology as a field of specialization was still in its infancy, however, a fact clearly noted by Henry Pancoast when he spoke before the First American Congress of Radiology in 1933. He stressed that in order to provide the best service possible it would be necessary to educate and train radiologists properly and, at the same time, to teach medical students and interns enough about radiology so that they would be able to make intelligent use of available radiological assistance. Furthermore, it was necessary to limit the practice of radiology to the medical profession to the exclusion of commercial laboratories, to cultivate an ethical role for the various radiological societies, and to create a board to certify specialists in the field.[93]

The precise, scientific nature of radiology was impressed upon interns who passed through the department in the 1930s. Although most remained for only two months, serving simultaneously on the Eye and Receiving Wards as well, many of them expressed interest in the present capabilities and potential for future development of radiology, particularly in new forms of treatment. The staff emphasized a broad, general knowledge to orient specialists in other fields comfortably and stressed both the capabilities and limitations of the radiological approach. Many interns were exposed for the first time to chronically ill patients while working in the therapy division and found this experience to be particularly helpful in their overall medical education. They were also generally impressed by the staff's medical expertise, especially outside their field of specialty.[94]

The introduction of interns and residents in the department in the 1920s initiated a profound change in the orientation of the teaching program, since staff members thus became responsible for individual, preceptor instruction to these graduates. At the same time staff members were beginning to spend more time on their own research projects, as residents became skilled enough to assume responsibility for some of the routine operation of the department. Students were also sometimes given special research projects, instead of or in addition to the routine work assignments. For example, Philip J. Hodes worked on a mammography project during his radiological rotation as an intern, learning the required techniques and then examining about 500 patients. This project proved so interesting that he decided to specialize in radiology.[95]

The interns had close to unilateral praise for the department's teaching program, and special mention was made of the willingness of the staff physicians to explain information in detail to the interns, as well as to explain what was and was not being seen, for example, in fluoroscopy sessions. Working in the department in conjunction with two other services meant that different interns spent varying amounts of time in radiology, so there was a considerable variation in the actual training that was received. Some preferred fluoroscopy, since it was thought likely that the individual physician might perform this procedure in his own office; others were particularly interested in therapy and the treatment program; and many aimed for as complete an overview as possible. Although the interns suffered definite scheduling difficulties, and many were unable to gain any exposure to some aspects of the specialty, the calibre of their instruction was nearly always praised.[96]

Although the department's staff was larger than it had been during the 1920s, including three or more staff physicians and a number of residents and rotating interns, it maintained an informality and congeniality in the interactions between the permanent and transient medical professionals. The staff's interest in teaching, and its cooperation and genuine friendliness, were emphasized repeatedly by interns on the service: "The radiographic and fluoroscopic work were extremely interesting and especially so, because of the time and pains spent discussing the interne's questions . . . . The spirit of fellowship and *esprit de corps* in the department I shall always remember."[97] Because there was such a limited number of Fellows, the residency training program was informal and tailored to the individual interests of each person. Radiology residents spent a portion of their time rotating through other departments in the hospital, and occasionally became involved in a research project while on one of these rotations in which they remained active for a considerable length of time. These outside interests were encouraged, and many worthwhile contributions to medical research were made by residents from the department.

By the early 1930s the residency program in radiology was a full two year course,[98] and the Fellows were gradually delegated responsibility for routine work in addition to their own research projects and teaching assignments. Accomodations were eventually found within the hospital to enable one of the Fellows to live there and be responsible for emergency work as it arose.[99] This arrangement replaced the interns on the hospital staff who had previously covered the department at night with the personal assistance of Dr. Pendergrass, who had always come in to take charge of the procedures.

Even though there was a very heavy workload for the physicians in the department, the overall operation was efficient, occasionally allowing them some flexibility in their schedules. Residents were, of course, expected to learn their specialty and to carry a share of the responsibility, but their constant presence was not always demanded in the department. The informality of the department at that time was recollected by Dr. Robert P. Barden, a resident during the mid-1930s:

[54]

I quickly discovered that the internes played tennis in the afternoons in the summer, therefore I played tennis almost every day that summer. First of all, there isn't a tennis court in the back of the University anymore. And secondly, the residents wouldn't be caught dead on the tennis court now, but it didn't seem to hurt anybody, I mean they still managed to learn and have some fun, so that's one little glimpse of the difference.[100]

It was during this period that Dr. Pendergrass actively worked to include a course in radiological physics in the department's educational offerings. As radiology gained nationwide acceptance it became increasingly evident that fully trained radiologists needed a good foundation in this area, and in 1934 Dr. S. Reid Warren, Jr., C. Justus Garrahan, Dallett B. O'Neill, and Charles E. Weyl began a series of lectures on the subject. This course was attended by physicians in the Department of Radiology and physicians in the Graduate School of Medicine, as well as outside physicians and student technicians. The physicists also taught special seminars for members of the Philadelphia Roentgen Ray Society.[101]

In 1932 the department began a School for X-ray Technicians to augment the supply of trained personnel in this field. In the early years the department's technical work had all been executed by physicians, with technicians merely assisting the doctors, although Drs. Pancoast and Pendergrass had employed one male technician during the 1920s who also performed some repairs on equipment. Generally Dr. Pancoast had insisted that each of his technicians also be a registered nurse. Student nurses had been rotated through the department, but as their curriculum expanded this rotation was eventually discontinued. Dr. Pendergrass felt it was a luxury to attempt to attract nurses to work as technicians, particularly since many women were concerned about exposure of the ovaries to radiation, so he suggeted that the department specifically train persons as technicians for future positions at University Hospital and at other institutions.

There was no precedent for this type of program. The department's approach combined both work experience and organized instruction. Residents were responsible for teaching anatomy, physiology, and some pharmacology, and the student technicians sat in on graduate courses in radiological physics. In later years the program became more structured, but in the early years instruction centered on practical experience, concentrating on fun-

[55]

damental procedures and on protection for both the operator and patient.[102]

The individual attention and atmosphere of genuine interest and concern, so strong in the teaching program, was also extended to the department's entire concept of service and patient care. It was a policy that each patient spoke personally to a physician, and students often accompanied staff members on the daily ward rounds which preceded diagnostic examinations and therapy treatments.[103]

The growth of the Department of Radiology was especially important because it incorporated a new emphasis on education and the delineation of a real scientific approach within the medical specialty, while maintaining its personal approach and real concern for both patients and students. Drs. Pancoast and Pendergrass were highly respected radiologists, destined to achieve unqualified recognition and acceptance within the University community; however, they were most concerned with their service to people.

Department Activity in the Early 1930s

There were still difficulties for the Department of Radiology during the early 1930s despite progress in achieving recognition as a specialty. Within the organizational structure of both the School of Medicine and University Hospital, the department operated as a subdivision of the Department of Surgery, creating administrative and financial headaches and maintaining a psychological barrier to the complete acceptance of radiology as an independent function.

The therapy division of the department was deeply in debt during this time, but Drs. Pancoast and Pendergrass felt a responsibility to treat the patients who came to the hospital, whether or not their funds were sufficient to cover the cost of their care. Most patients, in fact, had spent their available savings on diagnostic work, and had little or nothing left to cover the expenses of therapy. The department underwrote the therapy operation with funds from the diagnostic division, however, and continued to serve an ever increasing number of chronically ill patients.[104]

The fully-affiliated staff remained small: Dr. Pancoast, Dr. Pendergrass, and, for six years from 1928 until 1934, Dr. Karl Kornblum. Despite the considerable assistance provided by residents, the entire responsibility for the operation of the department was left to these men. Research work was continued throughout these years, but such work usually occurred after hours, when the day's routine duties were completed.

There was no sharp distinction between training for diagnostic and therapeutic radiology, and although the work was divided for administrative purposes the staff physicians were generalists, assigned varying duties. Not a great deal was known about radiation therapy, and for a considerable period of time the department's reputation stemmed from its diagnostic advances. Dr. Philip J. Hodes was head of the therapy division from 1936 until World War II, and as he recalled the operation: ". . . radiation therapy was being done, but a great deal of emphasis was not placed upon it because little was known about radiation therapy. As a matter of fact, soon after I finished my residency I was placed in charge of radiation therapy, which gives you an idea of how little I knew."[105]

Cramped facilities and a lack of radium seriously hampered the progress of the department at the beginning of the decade,[106] and the only physical expansion during these years involved the construction of a new darkroom in 1935.[107] New techniques were developed and implemented, and the patient load did not plunge too dramatically during the Depression, but the adverse financial climate did slow down the department's growth.

Some new therapy equipment was installed during the early 1930s, including a deep therapy unit to replace the one given by Mr. and Mrs. Caleb F. Fox in 1923. Another new unit was purchased in 1935, and with the addition of a machine to administer superficial therapy, the department had three pieces of new apparatus for its therapy operation.[108] In 1934 Dr. Floyd E. Keene, the physician who raised the money in 1930 to replace the original deep therapy unit, placed 100 milligrams of radium at the disposal of the department for use when it was not otherwise needed to treat patients by the staff of the Department of Gynecology. This gift raised the department's supply of radium to approximately one-half gram.[109]

During these years the department operated efficiently, and though small, its staff accomplished a great deal of work, generated considerable research, and expanded its education program

[57]

within a confined space and with somewhat limited equipment. Although the department was firmly established nationally and internationally, and its staff members continued to be instrumental in the coordination of national radiological activities, neither the School of Medicine nor University Hospital was convinced of its importance as a completely independent activity.

Pendergrass's and Pancoast's Departure Plans

By the mid-1930s Eugene Pendergrass's national reputation was so established that he received invitations to chair Departments of Radiology at both the University of Michigan and the University of Wisconsin. He visited these institutions, but was seriously concerned about the prospects for financing from the state legislatures of the respective states and, largely for that reason, turned down the two offers.

Shortly thereafter he received an invitation to head the department at Temple University in Philadelphia, and to design an entirely new installation for that operation, which he decided to accept. Pendergrass designed a new Department of Radiology for Good Samaritan Hospital, then the teaching hospital of Temple University, as well as a department in the medical school itself. The latter was physically located between the Department of Anatomy and the Department of Pathology, and presented an outstanding opportunity for cooperative teaching and research. Dr. Pancoast planned to join Dr. Pendergrass at Temple in 1940, following his retirement from Pennsylvania.

Several months before Dr. Pendergrass was to leave for Temple, however, Dr. Pancoast suffered a small stroke, and for the first time the University of Pennsylvania began to consider the question of a successor to Dr. Pancoast. The position was offered to Dr. Pendergrass, but he had already accepted Temple's invitation and was therefore placed in a particularly difficult position.

Eugene Pendergrass was actually more enthusiastic about staying at Pennsylvania where he could carry on the ideals and goals set by Dr. Pancoast, and the Dean at Temple graciously understood this. Dr. Pendergrass promised Dean Parkinson that he would find a replacement to head the department at Temple; after consultation with a number of prominent radiologists he recommended Dr. W. Edward Chamberlain, Professor of Radiology at Stanford University. Dr. Chamberlain was contacted, came to Philadelphia for an interview, saw the newly constructed department designed by Dr. Pendergrass, and accepted the position.[110]

Dr. Pancoast never completely regained his health after the stroke, and did not resume full responsibility for the day-to-day operation of the department. Dr. Pendergrass was appointed Professor of Radiology in 1936, and had already accepted the responsibility for short- and long-term planning in the department as well as for its routine activities.[111]

Initial Contacts with William Henry Donner

Eugene Pendergrass began to plan ahead during these years, contemplating programs which might prove feasible at a later date. He became involved in a project to develop X-ray equipment which would produce identical images at sea level and several thousand feet above sea level, to enable radiologists to determine standard appearances of the human anatomy on X-ray film, and persuaded the Moore School of Electrical Engineering and the Johnson Foundation of Medical Physics to lend assistance. In his search for funding for this project Dr. Pendergrass contacted William Henry Donner, a well-known philanthropist and head of the International Cancer Foundation.

William Henry Donner established the International Cancer Foundation in 1932, in memory of his son Joseph, who had died of cancer three years earlier, at the age of 35. Until the end of his life Donner devoted time to philanthropic causes, and his interest in cancer research supported scientists all over the world. His association with University Hospital's Department of Radiology was to be a natural outgrowth of this concern.[112]

Dr. Pendergrass explained his apparatus design project to Mr. Donner, who eventually offered to finance the Department of Radiology's portion of the work, but not the work in the Moore School or the Johnson Foundation. Dr. Pendergrass thanked him for his interest, but declined the funding, knowing that he could not obtain the necessary matching contributions. This association, however, was to be sustained.

Late in 1935 Mr. Donner called Dr. Pendergrass and asked him whether he knew anything about Chaoul therapy, a new approach to contact therapy devised by a German physician. Dr. Pendergrass had read about the procedure and had been so interested that, after reading a translation of an article by Dr. Chaoul, he had gone to Atlantic City to see an exhibit of the apparatus at the International Cancer Congress. Dr. Pendergrass was optimistic about the potential for this new procedure and intended to investigate it in much greater depth.

Mr. Donner told him that he had given Chaoul therapy units to two physicians in New York City, but that neither was particularly interested in this type of treatment. Dr. Pendergrass's enthusiasm motivated Donner to suggest that he might be able to give him one of the units in New York. He called shortly thereafter to ask Dr. Pendergrass to go to Europe to see the apparatus in operation, and to speak to Dr. Chaoul. Pendergrass was too busy to go. He planned to send an Associate, Dr. George W. Chamberlain, but after persuasion by the University's Vice President for Medical Affairs, Dr. and Mrs. Pendergrass found themselves on their way to Europe. The Pendergrasses spent several weeks abroad, during which time they visited Dr. Chaoul and a number of other physicians in Germany and England. By the completion of the trip Dr. Pendergrass was fully trained in the operation of the Chaoul apparatus, and aware of its potential; in March, 1936, after his return from abroad, the department received its Chaoul therapy unit.

Dr. Pendergrass's conscientious approach to the Chaoul therapy episode, and his economy while abroad, convinced Mr. Donner of his efficiency and dedication to the field of radiology. Thus began a long and cordial friendship. Mr. Donner was to make many generous contributions to the department and the University. Throughout these years he relied on Eugene Pendergrass as an expert authority and consulted him repeatedly for advice concerning the donation of X-ray apparatus to other institutions.[113]

Anticipation of Future Development: 1936–37

Dr. Pendergrass's promotion to the rank of Professor and his designation as "Chairman-elect" set the stage for long term development and expansion. A portion of the department was redesigned in 1936, to accomodate the installation of the Chaoul therapy unit and a 200 kilovolt shock-proof deep therapy unit. These machines doubled the capacity of the treatment division of the department and accounted for a considerable increase in the patient load during that year. Diagnostic work also increased considerably in 1936, as X-ray procedures were expanded to include the examination of patients for more disease conditions than ever before.[114]

An especially important research project was underway at this time: investigating the small intestine. This was one of the first studies of this organ, and the department worked in close cooperation with the gastrointestinal section of the Medical Clinic. With some assistance from the Departments of Surgical Research and Biochemistry in the School of Medicine, the department conducted a series of studies and received awards for the subsequent exhibit of the results at a number of medical and radiological society meetings.[115]

The patient load decreased somewhat by mid-1937, reflecting the national business conditions, but the facilities of the department continued crowded and taxed to their utmost. William Henry Donner's interest continued, and in the fall of 1936 he donated an ionization chamber to determine the dose distribution produced by the Chaoul therapy unit and a generating voltmeter to determine the secondary voltage of a number of pieces of equipment, probably the only one of its kind in the city.[116]

Mr. Donner's contributions satisfied pressing needs. Other additions were a rotating anode radiographic table, three new X-ray therapy tubes, and a filter device to be installed on the new deep therapy unit. The old photographic room was remodeled to permit a more efficient filing system, but the department was as yet unable to implement a master plan for reorganization and renovation. By early 1937 the staff was hopeful that plans for a completely new installation might be forthcoming, and everyone was thinking seriously of a new facility. Anticipating these future developments, the staff made small, urgently needed changes and additions, and waited.[117]

William Henry Donner's Bicentennial Contribution

In early 1938, William Henry Donner made a contribution of $200,000 to the Department of Radiology, in honor of his deceased son, William Henry Donner, Jr. The gift, although credited toward the University's Bicentennial Fund ending in 1940, was put to immediate use, and offered the department the opportunity to make immediate improvements as well as to plan for an entirely new installation.

Initial expenditures enabled the department to replace much of its old diagnostic and therapeutic apparatus with new, shock-proof equipment. The fluoroscopic rooms were remodeled, and new tables were installed, equipped for both routine radiographic work and fluoroscopic procedures. A radiographic unit designed especially for examinations of the head was also installed, as was a unit for laminography, enabling the physician to obtain an exposure of a special, localized area in any portion of the body, at any depth desired.

Mr. Donner's contribution additionally enabled the installation of new therapy apparatus, ". . . probably without peer in this country."[118] Two 200 kilovolt shock-proof units and a 135 kilovolt shock-proof superficial unit replaced the old therapy equipment, and, with the Chaoul treatment unit, provided highly sophisticated apparatus for the department's operation. The efficiency and convenience of the new machines enabled the staff to accommodate more patients each day, under circumstances considerably more pleasant than was formerly the case. New tube heads, of a unique construction, allowed ranges in target-to-surface distances that had been previously unattainable.

Teaching equipment was also added in 1938, and a projectoscope was purchased which projected a magnified view of an ordinary radiogram onto a screen, enabling an entire audience to see the film simultaneously and to discuss the case easily.

During this re-equipping process, the department enlisted the aid of Dr. S. Reid Warren and Mr. Dallett B. O'Neill from the Moore School of Electrical Engineering to advise them on the purchase of specific pieces of apparatus; at this time and in later years these two men offered much valuable advice.[119]

Additional apparatus was purchased in 1939, including a table for breast radiography and one adapted for ventriculography.

The purchase of three rotating anode tubes provided the capability to make rapid exposures of the spine, esophagus, and urinary tract, thereby expanding the diagnostic procedures available for analysis of these areas.[120]

A portion of Mr. Donner's gift was earmarked for the reinstallation of the department in the new Dulles-Agnew Wing of the hospital, under construction at this time. Donner himself officiated at the groundbreaking ceremonies for the new wing in December, 1939; the Agnew Pavilion replaced the old building of the same name which was destroyed by a fire in 1937, and the Dulles Pavilion, named in memory of a victim of the Titanic disaster, was built to the south and west of the Agnew Pavilion in a reversed "L" shape.[121]

Anticipation of the move to the new facility designed specially to meet the needs of the ever growing department eliminated the necessity to further remodel the White Building facility. A portion of the Donner gift continued to be spent on apparatus which would later be moved into the new facility, however. In 1940 these purchases included: new cones for use in therapy, equipment to permit rapid serial films to study the cardiovascular system, and a variety of other devices which enabled the convenient and efficient use of diagnostic equipment.[122]

The importance of Mr. Donner's gift cannot be overestimated because it enabled the department to replace its apparatus and to create a new physical installation all within a short period of time. The opportunity reinforced the department's reputation and was strong evidence of the calibre of an operation which could generate such interest and funding.

Cooperative Research:
Work for the Air Hygiene Foundation of America

In 1938 the Department of Radiology, in conjunction with the Moore School X-Ray Laboratory, undertook a major analysis of the methods of chest roentgenography available for use in industry. The study was sponsored by the Air Hygiene Foundation. Dr. Pendergrass was the principal radiological investigator, and Professor Charles Weyl, Dr. S. Reid Warren and Mr. Dallett B.

O'Neill were the principal technical investigators from the Moore School. Darrow E. Haagenson, a graduate electrical engineer, was hired to conduct many of the studies.

Increased awareness by employers of preventive measures to minimize occupational disease hazards was beginning to lead to expanded use of physical examinations at this time, both prior to and periodically during employment. The roentgen examination of the chest, a particularly important aspect of this procedure, was expensive when undertaken on a large scale, so the initial research on the project involved the analysis of exposure quality of roentgenograms made on film, and those made on specially prepared, sensitized paper, for industrial survey use. Major X-ray equipment manufacturers made available apparatus, darkroom facilities, roentgenographic paper, X-ray film, and developing chemicals for the investigations. The completed exposures were circulated to nearly fifty radiologists for quality analysis. The roentgenographic exposures made on paper were considerably inferior to those on film, but were considered acceptable for survey purposes in situations where patients with questionable diagnoses would receive more extensive examination.[123]

In later years the research concentrated specifically on silicosis and other occupational diseases caused by dust particles in the lungs. Dr. Eliot R. Clark of the Department of Anatomy joined the investigative team.[124] The Department of Radiology had been involved in work with these lung diseases ever since Dr. Pancoast's initial work in 1916, but this cooperative research venture was a unique opportunity to investigate disease symptoms as shown on different types of exposures, as well as to analyze the comparative technical merits of different methods of examination.

The research for the Air Hygiene Foundation was phased out as the United States entered World War II and a number of the investigators became involved in other projects. The work proved to be of particular importance, however, because the Armed Forces also adopted wide scale chest examination procedures for their recruits. Their primary interest was to diagnose men suffering from tuberculosis, and it was hoped that these precautionary actions would reduce the ultimate cost to the government in medical care and pensions. This consideration was equally valid for occupational diseases in industry.[125]

The Department of Radiology's reputation was clearly evident in the calibre of the cooperative research investigations in which it participated, and Eugene Pendergrass's expertise, combined with his enthusiasm for such joint investigations, would serve as the catalyst for the department's future efforts.

The Department Under New Leadership—1939

Henry Khunrath Pancoast died in May, 1939, and at that time Eugene Percival Pendergrass officially became Chairman of the Department of Radiology. The change in leadership caused no dramatic transition, since Dr. Pancoast had never regained his health sufficiently to reassume complete responsibility and Dr. Pendergrass had been running the operation for several years. Dr. Pancoast's death did, however, necessitate some organizational changes in the relationships between the University, the hospital, and the department.

The Department of Radiology had functioned as a subdivision of the Department of Surgery ever since Dr. Leonard began making exposures in 1896, and there was no change in this organizational structure during Henry Pancoast's time. Dr. Pancoast's reminiscences about his lifelong work in the department, published in February, 1938, made peripheral allusions to difficulties arising from this situation and emphasized another difficult problem facing radiologists during the 1930s: national recognition of their field of study as an independent specialization within the field of medicine, rather than as a merely technical operation. He emphasized the fact that it was often easier for a hospital to establish fees for radiological operations than to control activities in specialities like surgery or internal medicine, and that hospitals frequently overlooked the fact that a major component in the analysis of their general capability often involved the calibre of the radiological services available.[126] Pancoast's solution to the difficulties of dealing with the hospital administration was to operate the department much like a private practice, even though it remained a subdivision of the Department of Surgery. When it was given independent status in 1939 (one of Dr. Pendergrass's stipulations for remaining at the University), Dr. Pendergrass continued to operate the department much as his predecessor had.

The department hired its own physicians, technicians, and

nurses, and they were paid on a salary scale determined by Dr. Pendergrass. The department received most of its income from private patients, although a portion of these fees was paid to the hospital. The hospital received all income from patients in the wards and from patients in the out-patient dispensaries. Income from the latter groups of patients was sporadic, though, since a great many individuals were unable to pay for their medical expenses; it was not until the Blue Cross system was established that the hospital received substantial income from out-patients. Expenses for the department's therapy operation were particularly high.

The hospital charged the Department of Radiology for the space which it occupied. This assessment included normal housekeeping services, and in some ways the department was treated as though it were renting space from the hospital. Most often the department purchased new equipment from its own income or with money from private contributions, and although it charged the hospital for films used on ward patients, it did not assess a fee for the processing of the films or for the doctors' and technicians' time. Costs of preparation for hospital seminars, particularly the time spent by the technicians who prepared the materials, were never reimbursed in the hospital-department finances.

The department's participation in the medical education program was extensive at this time, but the funding it received from the School of Medicine was minimal. Even after the department achieved independent status its budget remained very small; the funding received was not enough to pay for all the slides necessary for the teaching program. The department's physicians did receive a contribution toward their salaries from the School of Medicine, but the contribution was exceedingly low relative to their teaching load.[127]

In light of the department's limited funding sources from the income generated by private patients, the contributions made by Mr. Donner and other individuals became even more significant. The only means to purchase large pieces of equipment, or to considerably expand the staff, was by developing the interest of potential donors and soliciting their support. Dr. Pendergrass successfully convinced Mr. Donner of the validity of the program at the University of Pennsylvania in the mid-1930s, and his subsequent Bicentennial contribution proved very important in the department's growth.

NOTES

1. Hospital of the University of Pennsylvania, *Annual Report of the Board of Managers* (30 June 1939), p. 14.

2. Henry K. Pancoast, "Reminiscences of a Radiologist," *American Journal of Roentgenology and Radium Therapy* **39**, No. 2 (1938): 172.

3. Hospital of the University of Pennsylvania, *Annual Report of the Board of Managers* (31 December 1902), p. 102.

4. Hospital of the University of Pennsylvania, *Annual Report of the Board of Managers* (31 August 1904), p. 129.

5. Hospital of the University of Pennsylvania, *Annual Report*, 1902, p. 102.

6. *Ibid.*

7. *Catalogue of the University of Pennsylvania, Fasciculus of the Department of Medicine* (Philadelphia: 1900–03).

8. Pancoast, "Reminiscences," p. 172.

9. Hospital of the University of Pennsylvania, *Annual Report of the Board of Managers* (31 December 1903), p. 117.
Pancoast, "Reminiscences," p. 182.

10. *Catalogue, Department of Medicine,* 1903–04, pp. 271, 273.

11. Hospital of the University of Pennsylvania, *Annual Report*, 1903, p. 54.

12. Hospital of the University of Pennsylvania, *Annual Report*, 1904, p. 18.
Hospital of the University of Pennsylvania, *Annual Report of the Board of Managers* (31 August 1905), p. 18.

13. Pancoast, "Reminiscences," p. 173.

14. Hospital of the University of Pennsylvania, *Annual Report*, 1904, p. 129.

15. Hospital of the University of Pennsylvania, *Annual Report*, 1903, p. 117.

16. Pancoast, "Reminiscences," p. 172.

17. *Ibid.,* p. 170.

18. Hospital of the University of Pennsylvania, *Annual Report*, 1904, p. 130.

19. Pancoast, "Reminiscences," p. 175.

20. "Convention of the American Roentgen Ray Society," *Old Penn,* 12 December 1903.

21. *Transactions of the Fourth Annual Meeting of the American Roentgen Ray Society, December 9–10, 1903* (Philadelphia: 1904).

22. *Ibid.,* p. 66.   23. *Ibid.,* pp. 153–54.

24. *Ibid.,* p. 155.   25. *Ibid.,* p. 175.

26. Hospital of the University of Pennsylvania, *Annual Report*, 1905, p. 133.

27. Hospital of the University of Pennsylvania, *Annual Report,* 1904, pp. 129–130.

28. *Ibid.,* p. 129.　　　　　　29. *Ibid.,* p. 130.

30. *Ibid.,* p. 13.

31. Mary V. Stephenson, *The First Fifty Years of the Training School for Nurses of the Hospital of the University of Pennsylvania* (Philadelphia: J. B. Lippincott Company, 1940), p. 102.

32. Hospital of the University of Pennsylvania, *Annual Report,* 1905, p. 133.

33. Stephenson, *School for Nurses,* pp. 102–03.

34. George E. Pfahler, "The Early History of Roentgenology in Philadelphia: The History of the Philadelphia Roentgen Ray Society, Part I: 1899–1920," *American Journal of Roentgenology, Radium Therapy and Nuclear Medicine* **75**, No. 1 (1956): 14–22.

35. Pancoast, "Reminiscences," p. 178.

36. Hospital of the University of Pennsylvania, *Annual Report of the Board of Managers* (31 August 1906), p. 131.

37. Pancoast, "Reminiscences," p. 181.

38. *Ibid.*

39. *Ibid.,* p. 183.

40. Hospital of the University of Pennsylvania, *Annual Report of the Board of Managers* (31 August 1909), p. 18.

41. *Scope* (Philadelphia: 1910), p. 63.

42. Trustees of the University of Pennsylvania, *Board Minutes* **15** (1911): 194.

43. Trustees of the Medico-Chirurgical College, *Board Minutes* (Philadelphia: n.d.): 319.

44. Hospital of the University of Pennsylvania, *Annual Report of the Board of Managers* (31 August 1911), p. 114.

45. *Catalogue, Department of Medicine,* 1911–12, p. 384.

46. *Scope,* p. 192.

47. Pancoast, "Reminiscences," p. 183.

48. Pfahler, "Early History of Roentgenology."

49. "Henry Khunrath Pancoast," *Radiology and Clinical Photography* **15**, No. 2 (1939).

50. Hospital of the University of Pennsylvania, *Annual Report,* 1905, p. 139.

51. Hospital of the University of Pennsylvania, *Annual Report of the Board of Managers* (30 June 1914), p. 21.

52. Hospital of the University of Pennsylvania, *Annual Report of the Board of Managers* (30 June 1915), p. 23.

53. Pancoast, "Reminiscences," p. 184.

54. Hospital of the University of Pennsylvania, *Annual Report,* 1915, p. 128.

55. Pancoast, "Reminiscences," p. 180.

56. Eugene P. Pendergrass, Personal Interview, 10 August 1976.

57. Hospital of the University of Pennsylvania, *Annual Report of the Board of Managers* (30 June 1917), p. 148.

58. Pancoast, "Reminiscences," p. 181.

59. Hospital of the University of Pennsylvania, *Annual Report of the Board of Managers* (30 June 1916), p. 135.

60. Pancoast, "Reminiscences," p. 182.

61. Hospital of the University of Pennsylvania, *Annual Report*, 1917, p. 22.

62. *Catalogue, Department of Medicine*, 1917–19, 1920–21.

63. University of Pennsylvania, *The University Bulletin: Graduate School of Medicine, 1919–20* (Philadelphia: 1919), pp. 30–31.

64. Pancoast, "Reminiscences," p. 185.

65. Hospital of the University of Pennsylvania, *Annual Report*, 1917, p. 16; Hospital of the University of Pennsylvania, *Annual Report of the Board of Managers* (30 June 1919), p. 18; Pendergrass, Personal Interview, 23 February 1976.

66. *Ibid.*

67. Pancoast, "Reminiscences," p. 185.

68. Pendergrass, Personal Interview, 23 February 1976.

69. *Ibid.*

70. Pancoast, "Reminiscences," pp. 184–85.

71. Pendergrass, Personal Interview, 23 February 1976.

72. *Ibid.*

73. *Ibid.*

74. Hospital of the University of Pennsylvania, *Annual Report of the Board of Managers* (30 June 1924), p. 19; Pendergrass, Personal Interview, 23 February 1976.

75. Stephenson, *School for Nurses*, p. 143.

76. Hospital of the University of Pennsylvania, *Annual Report of the Board of Managers* (30 June 1923), p. 25.

77. Hospital of the University of Pennsylvania, *Annual Report*, 1924, p. 23.

78. Hospital of the University of Pennsylvania, *Annual Report of the Board of Managers* (30 June 1925), p. 26.

79. Henry K. Pancoast to Board of Managers, Hospital of the University of Pennsylvania, 5 January 1921, Document Box.

80. Pancoast, "Reminiscences," p. 185.

81. Pendergrass, Personal Interview, 23 February 1976.

82. Hospital of the University of Pennsylvania, *Annual Report of the Board of Managers* (30 June 1926), p. 23.

83. Hospital of the University of Pennsylvania, *Annual Report of the Board of Managers* (30 June 1927), p. 26.

84. Hospital of the University of Pennsylvania, *Annual Report of the Board of Managers* (30 June 1928), p. 27.

85. Hospital of the University of Pennsylvania, *Annual Report of the Board of Managers* (30 June 1929), p. 25.

86. Hospital of the University of Pennsylvania, *Annual Report,* 1928, p. 22.

87. S. Reid Warren, Jr., "Notes on Electromedical Work in the Moore School of Electrical Engineering, University of Pennsylvania, 24 July 1964"; S. Reid Warren, Jr., Personal Interview, 25 February 1976.

88. Pancoast, "Reminiscences," p. 184.

89. *Ibid.*

90. Hospital of the University of Pennsylvania, *Annual Report of the Board of Managers* (30 June 1931), p. 32.

91. Pendergrass, Personal Interview, 11 August 1976.

92. Hospital of the University of Pennsylvania, *Annual Report,* 1931, p. 23; Trustees of the University of Pennsylvania, *Board Minutes* **20** (1930): 387.

93. Percy Brown, "Henry Khunrath Pancoast—An Appreciation," *American Journal of Roentgenology and Radium Therapy* **38**, No. 1 (1937): 4–10.

94. Department of Radiology, Hospital of the University of Pennsylvania, Interne's Register.

95. Philip J. Hodes, Taped Comments, Winter 1976.

96. Department of Radiology, Interne's Register.

97. *Ibid.*, "Comments of George C. Ham (1937)," p. 90.

98. Hospital of the University of Pennsylvania, *Annual Report,* 1931, p. 32.

99. *Ibid.*, p. 33.

100. Robert P. Barden, Personal Interview, 16 March 1976.

101. Warren, "Electromedical Work," p. 1.

102. Pendergrass, Personal Interview, 13 August 1976.

103. Pendergrass, Personal Interview, 11 August 1976.

104. Pendergrass, Personal Interview, 17 June 1976.

105. Hodes, Taped Comments, Winter 1976.

106. Hospital of the University of Pennsylvania, *Annual Report,* 1931, p. 32.

107. Hospital of the University of Pennsylvania, *Annual Report of the Board of Managers* (31 May 1935), p. 8.

108. Pancoast, "Reminiscences," p. 185.

109. *Ibid.*

110. Pendergrass, Personal Interview, 17 June 1976.

111. Hospital of the University of Pennsylvania, *Annual Report of the Board of Managers* (31 May 1937), p. 12.

112. Biographical Information of William Henry Donner, 1864–1953, Research Files, Donner Center and Foundation, Hospital of the University of Pennsylvania.

113. Pendergrass, Personal Interview, 17 June 1976.

114. Hospital of the University of Pennsylvania, *Annual Report of the Board of Managers* (31 May 1936), p. 64.

115. *Ibid.*, p. 85.

116. Hospital of the University of Pennsylvania, *Annual Report,* 1937, pp. 68–69.

117. *Ibid.*, pp. 69–70.

118. Hospital of the University of Pennsylvania, *Annual Report of the Board of Managers* (31 May 1938), p. 72.

119. *Ibid.*

120. Hospital of the University of Pennsylvania, *Annual Report,* 1939, p. 70.

121. Hospital of the University of Pennsylvania, *Annual Report of the Board of Managers* (31 May 1940), p. 9.

122. *Ibid.*, pp. 68–69.

123. Air Hygiene Foundation of America, Inc., *The Comparative Values of Chest Roentgenograms Made on Film and on Paper for Industrial Surveys,* Medical Series, Bulletin No. II (Pittsburgh: 1939), pp. 15–16.

124. Hospital of the University of Pennsylvania, *Annual Report,* 1939, p. 70; Hospital of the University of Pennsylvania, *Annual Report,* 1940, p. 60; Hospital of the University of Pennsylvania, *Annual Report of the Board of Managers* (31 May 1941), p. 68.

125. Eugene P. Pendergrass, S. Reid Warren, and D. E. Haagensen, *A Comparison of Stereoscopic Miniature Chest Films, Single Roentgenograms on Paper, and Single Roentgenograms on Large Films,* Medical Series, Bulletin No. V (Pittsburgh: 1942), p. 1.

126. Pancoast, "Reminiscences," pp. 169–70.

127. Pendergrass, Personal Interview, 4 April 1976.

THE PENDERGRASS ERA
1940–1960

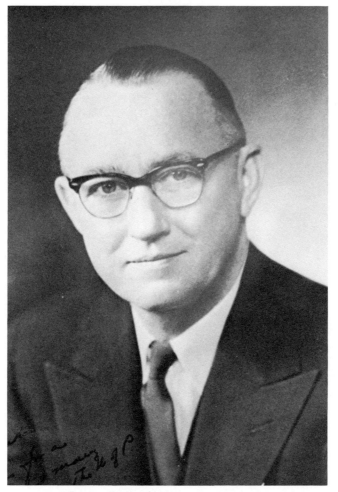

Eugene P. Pendergrass, 1937–1961

Departmental Operations in the
Early Years of World War II

The department continued to grow and expand in the years following Dr. Pendergrass's assumption of the duties of Chairman,
and plans for the new facility promised to provide the highest
possible quality. While awaiting its completion the department
operated under extremely crowded conditions, but morale was
high due to the considerable increase in apparatus and the awareness of imminent improvements.

Despite uncomfortable areas in the department's White Building location, no alterations were made to the space after 1937,
since the staff anticipated moving to the new Dulles Building
early in 1942. A gift of a periscope for treating cancer of the cervix
was received in 1941. This instrument was especially appreciated
because it had been designed by a former student in the department, Dr. Percy D. Hay, Jr.[1]

As national research progressed on the cyclotron, Dr. Pendergrass became very interested in building one for the department.
In 1940 Mr. Donner began a fund for the purchase of a cyclotron.[2]
Dr. Pendergrass had already spent time in Berkeley with Drs.
Ernest Lawrence and Robert Stone, where he learned about the
medical application of cyclotrons. After returning to Philadelphia, he successfully encouraged Mr. Donner to go to California
to meet these gentlemen and see their work first hand. Mr. Donner was asked for funds to construct a building for Dr. Lawrence
while there, and he agreed to provide the necessary sum.

Mr. Donner was still most interested in providing the funds for
a cyclotron at Pennsylvania, however, being particularly impressed with the Department of Radiology's qualifications to
carry on this sort of research after speaking with the specialists
in California. Dr. Pendergrass began to recruit the necessary staff
and to develop plans for the cyclotron's location. Application was
made for the necessary metals, but due to the war effort most,
particularly copper, were in short supply. Some time after the
initiation of the project Dr. Thomas S. Gates, President of the
University of Pennsylvania, received a call from the Secretary of
State requesting that he convince Dr. Pendergrass to drop the

project for this reason. The department remained interested in the cyclotron, but quickly became involved in a number of other projects so that by the time metals would have been available, the staff's activities were directed elsewhere.[3]

The training course for radiologic technicians improved during these years, and applications to enter the program increased so greatly that the department was able to elevate its entrance requirements.[4] The number of students was increased in 1941, and the curriculum made more comprehensive.[5]

The *esprit de corps* and warmth exuded by the department's staff toward patients, students, and visitors made the Department of Radiology one of the most respected in the hospital service. The atmosphere was noted by outsiders, and reiterated over and again by students and physicians who spent time there during their terms of service in the hospital. One intern commented that his reaction was one of ". . . genuine appreciation for the consideration shown by the entire staff and personnel as to instruction, advice and appointments . . ."[6] while another exphasized the "excellent personnel, and spirit in the department. . . ."[7] The hard work caused by the increasing patient load and the difficulties of working in constrained areas were made easier by everyone's cooperative attitudes. One enthusiastic intern was particularly vivid in his description of the service: ". . . this department is certainly one of the most outstanding in [the] world for equipment and personnel and it is only natural that young men would like to profit in the utmost from the association."[8]

Move to the New Department—March, 1942

Progress in the new installation in the Dulles Building was slow, but the department was able to move into the facility in March, 1942. The space had been specially designed to accomodate private and clinic patients, had ample room for diagnostic, therapeutic, and research activities, and included a sophisticated film processing system. The building was shaped like the letter "T," with the stem part housing diagnostic apparatus and the crosspiece the therapeutic apparatus. There were separate entrances for private and clinic patients, and in some cases separate examination rooms. Private patients also had a room in which to wait. The film

processing system was located in the middle of the building between parallel corridors that served private and clinic patients,
and was conveniently accessible from either area. The basement
provided permanent film storage space.

The department's ultramodern film processing center was especially impressive. In this facility films were handled in baskets,
instead of individually, to speed the developing process and to
minimize scratches due to handling. The dryers, specially designed by members of the staff, were located in the wall between
the processing room and the film files, and could be adjusted to
change both their capacity and the length of drying time. The
overall system incorporated the most up-to-date equipment
available, and substantially simplified the entire developing process.[9]

Although eventual expansion in the White Building had
created a centralized area for therapeutic work, the move to the
new facility in the Dulles Building was especially significant because it was the first time that the design included a comprehensive therapy area. Upon final installation in the new building, the
department was able once again to emphasize its comprehensive
services and to assert that the new facility would "... bring credit
to the Hospital of the University of Pennsylvania."[10]

Departmental Operations in the New Facility

The department was very proud of its convenient new facility
that was opened during the war years, despite difficulties due to
the fact that the move to the new installation occurred simultaneously with the departure of several staff members for military
service. The expansion of available services and the resulting
increase in the patient load made especially heavy demands on
the staff members who remained in Philadelphia.

Eugene Pendergrass was offered and accepted the position of
Radiologist to the European Theater for the United States Army,
but University Hospital would not release him for military service. In his place he recommended Kenneth A. Allen, a Denver
radiologist who had worked with him as an intern during the
1920s. Allen developed a highly successful program.[11]

A number of staff members from the department left Philadelphia with the 20th General Unit, the University Hospital medical unit which served in India during the war. Within a period of a few months in 1942 the department lost seven physicians, including the two experienced staff radiologists who had worked with Dr. Pendergrass. Philip Hodes went to India with the University Hospital Unit, and George Chamberlain transferred to the Reading Hospital. Pendergrass persuaded Dr. Robert P. Barden, a department Fellow during the mid-1930s, to return to the department from Episcopal Hospital in Philadelphia. These two men continued the operation of the department with the assistance of a single experienced technician. In addition to their routine clinical duties the physicians were ultimately responsible for the complete educational program, training residents, medical students, and student technicians. Dr. S. Reid Warren continued as a consultant and worked as the department physicist. With his help, the assistance of some other consultants, and the aid of a group of residents who quickly assumed responsibility, the department continued to function smoothly.[12]

This smooth operation of the department did not come about easily, however. The experienced staff could only extend itself so far, and even after Dr. Karl Kornblum, a staff member in the late 1920s, returned to work in the department half-time in 1942, the senior men were under considerable pressure. Most of the films were read by residents in the department, although unusual ones were put aside so that Dr. Pendergrass or Dr. Barden could look at them at a later time.[13] In order to finish all their work, physicians remained in the department reading films until late in the evening and worked both Saturday and Sunday as well. Drs. Barden and Kornblum shared responsibility for the department's fluoroscopy on alternate weeks, heading a team that included a physician, two technicians, and two student technicians.[14] Dr. Pendergrass retained primary responsibility for the therapy program following Dr. Hodes's departure, although Dr. Barden was also somewhat involved in this aspect of the department's work. Fellows rotated through the diagnosis and therapy divisions, and coverage was always arranged so that there was one experienced resident in therapy.[15] The department continued to train technicians, but even with this program there was a shortage of technical personnel to assist with all the programs.[16] The staff had little time to participate in seminars or to prepare exhibits for radiological meetings, and their own research projects were relegated to the late evening hours.[17]

[78]

A portion of the department's increased patient load was due to an expansion in diagnostic services. During this time the department assumed responsibility for a number of comprehensive surveys, including annual chest examinations for each nurse and intern on the staff at University Hospital, as well as for all the Visiting Nurses in Philadelphia. The staff also began a program of chest examinations of all women who visited the hospital for prenatal care; this marked the implementation of a long-range program to examine the chests of each patient visiting the hospital, whether as an in-patient or an out-patient.[18]

With the expanded capabilities of the therapy program in the new installation, the Department of Radiology began to function at its maximum daily capacity level, treating approximately fifty patients each day.[19] Dr. Hodes's departure had created supervisory personnel problems, and although Fellows generally ran the routine operation, there were serious problems regarding the summer months. In the summer of 1943, a decision was made to close the therapy operation completely for the month of August,[20] but after considerable discussion and rescheduling the decision was reversed, and the therapeutic activities continued without a break.[21] The mere consideration of such a drastic measure indicates the difficult conditions under which the staff was operating.

Despite an ever increasing patient load, the Department of Radiology continued to work on cooperative research projects with other departments in the University. In 1941 Drs. Gaylord P. Harnwell and Louis N. Ridenour, Professors of Physics, presented the department with a radium measuring device and provided valuable help on therapeutic difficulties. Dr. Warren and Mr. O'Neill from the Moore School continued to provide assistance to the radiologists, particularly regarding the purchase of more equipment for the new installation in the Dulles Building.[22] Beginning about 1943 the Department of Radiology also expanded its research to include work in orthopedics and became increasingly close to the hospital's Orthopedic Department. An orthopedist spent time in the Department of Radiology each day reading films, and once a week the two departments held a joint conference to analyze particularly interesting cases.[23]

As was the case with World War I, during these years the department offered a variety of courses geared toward training members of the Armed Forces. General refresher courses were offered, designed specifically for radiologists, sometimes in conjunction with programs organized by other departments in the hospital. One interdepartmental program, six weeks in length, was specially organized for physicians in the Army and included work in maxillofacial surgery, thoracic surgery, and surgery of the extremities, in addition to the study of radiologic techniques and diagnosis. The Navy sent personnel, generally not physicians, to the Department of Radiology for two months of intensive training in the fundamentals of radiologic technique. These men functioned in the capacity of X-ray technicians. The department's staff also participated in "Wartime Graduate Training," an organized series of refresher courses, generally in the format of lectures and panel discussions, for servicemen stationed at nearby locations.[24]

The department's operation during the war years was further complicated by shortages, and in some cases rationing, of both X-ray tubes and X-ray film. The film supply became critically low at times, forcing the staff to borrow films from other hospitals or exercise influence within the Armed Forces structure to secure badly needed films.[25] The film shortage was understandable: prior to the war ninety percent of the available national supply had been used in medicine, whereas during the war the Army and Navy used twenty-five percent of the total supply and industry utilized another twenty-five percent, leaving nonmilitary medical installations in the country without sufficient supplies to make unlimited diagnostic exposures.[26]

When the installation in the Dulles Building was completed, the department possessed the very latest in modern apparatus, including advanced therapy equipment and diagnostic apparatus to execute almost any examination with dispatch.[27] The original plans had called for expansion to include a cyclotron, but following the delay of that project due to material shortages and military needs, the department changed the focus of its plans for growth and instead decided to expand the therapy operation to include a million-volt unit.

This unit was specially designed and built by the Westinghouse Company for the department and was unique because a special gas insulation system enabled it to be more economically packaged than a conventional million-volt unit. After the apparatus had been built and paid for, however, the government discovered that its oscillations would scramble German broadcasts, and at the request of a number of high-level government officials, the department released the unit for the war effort. It was installed in northern Scotland and enabled the Allies to interrupt the German broadcasting which had been disturbing much of England, Wales, and Scotland.[28]

Following the release of the million-volt unit, the department reconsidered its plans once again, and in early 1943 the decision was made to acquire a 400 kilovolt unit and a betatron. Mr. Donner's contributions had been responsible for the financing of these planned acquisitions from the start, and in March, upon receipt of his approval, the department attempted to acquire the two new pieces of apparatus.[29] However, no 400 kilovolt therapy machines were available at the time, though one manufacturing firm thought that it could make one for the department, nor were there any commercial betatron models available.[30] The 400 kilovolt unit was eventually installed, but this early delay, and the general expenditure of time and frustration, taxed the staff's energy.

Dr. Pendergrass and the rest of the staff kept in close touch with staff members in the Armed Forces and each staff member was kept on the payroll, the department paying the balance between his or her military salary and the salary which he or she would have received in Philadelphia. Despite increases in the staff to replace those members in the military, Dr. Pendergrass promised that everyone's job would be retained, and after the war most personnel were reabsorbed into the department's operation.[31]

The team effort and *esprit de corps* among the department's staff helped it to pull through several difficult war years. Shortages in personnel and equipment, and disappointments regarding new purchases of apparatus, presented psychological as well as practical obstacles to the operation, yet the staff continued to function effectively, to pursue individual interests, and to offer increased services to patients. The expansion might have been smoother without war shortages, but with the constant support of their Chief, the staff operated a first-rate department and continued its reputation for excellence.

Dr. Pendergrass's Participation
in the Atomic Bomb Program

Although he was unable to go to Europe to serve in that theater during the war, Eugene Pendergrass was commissioned in both the Army and Navy from 1946 until 1948, and served as a Radiation Safety Officer during the testing programs that followed the explosion of the nuclear warheads over Japan. He was assigned to a large group responsible for analyzing and predicting the results of exposure to radioactivity and served with a number of other scientists and radiologists.

Pendergrass's portion of the project was under the direction of Dr. Stafford Warren, Professor of Radiology at the University of Rochester. After indoctrination, the group was sent to an island in the South Pacific where some 80,000 Americans, including specialists in every aspect of science, were gathered to carry out this research. Classes were held each day, and lecturers did their best to hypothesize the long range effects of radiation exposure. Dr. Pendergrass's primary responsibility was to warn people when and how to protect themselves. As a physician, he was also responsible for general medical work and became involved in some counseling situations as well. There was real concern among many of the servicemen about their safety on this operation, and Pendergrass found the chaplains and priests especially helpful in allaying fear among the men.

Pendergrass was most directly involved during the series of underwater detonations of the atomic bomb. A number of Navy vessels were deserted, tightly sealed, near the test site, and it was his responsibility to analyze the degree of contamination following the explosions. Results showed a surprisingly high degree of radioactivity. Pendergrass and his associates were repeatedly exposed to considerable amounts of radiation, but not a single individual suffered permanent damage.

After a few months Dr. Warren was required to return to the United States, so Dr. Pendergrass was in complete charge of the operation for a time. He was in the South Pacific for close to six months in 1946, and was also made a consultant to the Atomic Bomb Casulty Commission when it was established in Tokyo, Hiroshima, and Nagasaki. He returned to Philadelphia shortly thereafter, but remained involved with the Commission as an interested, though distant, consultant.[32]

Emphases of the Educational Program in the 1940s

The department's staff was involved in teaching on a myriad of levels: undergraduate medical students, graduate medical students, interns, residents, student technicians, and physicians from other institutions. The approach combined both formal and didactic instruction, and there was considerable personal interaction with the staff members.

The teaching program for undergraduate medical students was rather limited during the 1940s, its scope much the same as it had been in the 1930s. As in the past, the first and second year students were introduced to the department, along with a number of other specialties, at clinical conferences. Practical exposure to radiology came only during the third year, and even that was limited.[33] Planned changes in the curriculum in the late 1940s would offer electives in radiology for the first time. Third year students would be able, possibly, to choose instruction in either diagnosis or radiation therapy. Students would also be encouraged to work in pathology or anatomy and combine that work with a project in radiology, and especially interested students could work with radio-isotopes. These curriculum changes were not implemented immediately but marked, for the first time, a real interest in undergraduate medical education.

Even before these opportunities for elective course work in radiology, however, medical students and graduate students in other fields had expressed interest in the specialty by working in the department during summers, or pursuing independent research projects during the academic year. Two medical students spent the summer of 1944 working in the department, and beginning in 1947 John Hale, a graduate student in electrical engineering, began to express an interest in the field and to work with the staff physicians and consultants from the Moore School.[34] He was later to become the department's first full-time radiological physicist.

Interns had been serving rotations in the department for nearly twenty-five years by the end of the 1940s when changes in the hospital's internship program necessitated concurrent changes in the department's scheduling of intern instruction. During the 1930s and early 1940s, interns had complained because their two month service in the Department of Radiology was shared with responsibilities in both the Eye and Receiving Wards. There was not a uniform exposure to the department's many programs, since interns spent varying amounts of time learning about the department's many functions. In 1949 the term of service was shortened, and the intern generally spent two weeks or less working solely in the Department of Radiology. The advantages of concentrating in one department were offset by the exceedingly short length of the service, and although the staff revamped the approach with an eye to the overall operation, the amount of practical experience was minimal.[35]

The department continued its program to train X-ray technicians throughout the 1940s, although at times during the war years it seemed likely that this program would be phased out. The curriculum became more extensive, the calibre of the students improved early in the decade, and by 1942 the teaching approach included practical demonstrations by other technicians and physicians as well as special classroom courses. During the 1930s the student technicians had joined the graduate physicians for Dr. Warren's course in radiological physics, but in the fall of 1942 he introduced a new physics course, taught specifically for the student technicians.[36] Staff physicians had considerable contact with these students and, in addition to demonstrating practical techniques, were responsible for weekly quiz sessions.[37] New classes of technicians began at sporadic intervals throughout the 1940s, and the students gained, through a combination of formal and preceptorial instruction, a thorough knowledge of X-ray technology.

The department's primary teaching emphasis was directed toward the group of physicians composed of Fellows and residents. At some times this semantic distinction was of particular importance (a Fellow might be a physician staying on after his residency for special work, or he might be receiving funding from a specific outside organization), but at other times the titles were used interchangeably. However, it was generally felt that the term "Fellow" carried more status throughout the hospital, and it was used as much as possible.

During the 1940s the fellowship program was three years in length and most of the physicians were also enrolled as degree candidates in the Graduate School of Medicine. Their initial exposure to the department included rotations through both the diagnostic and therapeutic divisions, and later often included rotations through other departments in the hospital as well. Fellows were enthusiastically encouraged to pursue independent research projects and were often asked to report on the progress of their work during staff meetings.

Dr. Pendergrass stressed the active participation of Fellows in the department's routine as soon as possible, and encouraged other staff members to allow residents to execute various techniques after a minimum of observation.[38] Fellows were also eventually assigned their own interns and were responsible for training them during their term of service in the department.[39]

Throughout their training in the department, the Fellows were treated as respected members of the professional team, and Dr. Pendergrass expected them to work just as hard as the rest of the staff. They worked in a supportive, non-competitive atmosphere, and their opinions were sought and listened to a staff meetings.[40] Dr. Pendergrass had the knack of encouraging these young physicians, knowing when to give them responsibility. Under this guidance they made effective contributions to the department's operation.

There was a definite emphasis on diagnostic training during this period, and although residents were exposed to the therapy program, it always took second place to the diagnostic side. This was particularly clear when Fellows were assigned to cover for doctors who were attending conferences, because the physicians on the treatment side always provided the necessary manpower to replace the absent doctor.[41] Residents were also responsible for staffing the department on evenings and weekends to provide necessary emergency coverage. Provisions were made for modest accommodations at the hospital for the physician on call,[42] and during these times this individual was responsible, with the assistance of a technician, for the department's complete operation.

The staff also encouraged the Fellows to spend a portion of their training outside the Department of Radiology, so residents rotated to other departments in the hospital or to other hospitals. Fellows often spent time in the Departments of Pathology, Surgery, and Surgical Research, and in 1949, for the first time, a resident rotated through the Department of Gynecology.

Interaction with the Department of Gynecology was particularly important because that department had been treating its patients with radium ever since 1917, with little or no input from the radiologists. Dr. Pancoast had originally suggested that Dr. John Clark, Chief of Gynecology, treat his own cancer patients, but subsequent lack of communication and cooperation meant that the gynecologists were working without any consultation on treatment programs or consideration of possible new techniques. When Dr. Pendergrass sent his first Fellow to the Department of Gynecology, he had him make radiographs after the insertion of radium in the vagina by the gynecologists. His results showed that in nearly eighty percent of the cases the radium slipped, making the treatment ineffective for treating cancer of the cervix, and potentially dangerous. Although initially upset, the gynecologists acknowledged their difficulty and began to send their residents to the Department of Radiology for training in various types of therapy. This exchange of residents proved very successful and was the beginning of a good cooperative relationship between the two departments.[43]

Residents were also sent on rotations to other hospitals to give them an opportunity to see radiology departments in different contexts, including community hospitals and rural institutions. Since a number of these physicians would not be practicing radiology in a large university setting with the special problems of an academic department, the rotation to other hospitals was a particularly important part of their general radiological training.

By the end of the 1940s Dr. Pendergrass had begun to secure outside funding to help finance the fellowship program. This was important because he was in the process of increasing the program's length to four years. The number of Fellows had increased dramatically following World War II, and this substantial increase in staff, without concurrent increases in departmental income, would have placed a heavy strain on the operating budget. Considerable funding came from the National Cancer Institute and the national and local branches of the American Cancer Society, in further recognition of the department's reputation and status in American radiology.

At about the same time the department was also given its first fellowship, by members of the Heublein family. Established in 1946, the Arthur Carl Heublein Memorial Fellowship was named in memory of an eminent radiologist from Hartford, Connecticut. His son, Gilbert W. Heublein, had trained as a radiologist under Dr. Pendergrass at Pennsylvania, and his association with the department was responsible for the establishment of the memorial to the senior Dr. Heublein at University Hospital.

Members of the Heublein family and Heublein, Inc., the family liquor company, established the original fund and contributed to it periodically. This fund was used to supplement the stipends of outstanding Fellows, and was important in later years because its unrestricted nature allowed the department to use it to support a number of foreign physicians who were ineligible for federally funded grants.

The department's extensive participation in educational programs was supplemented by programs for practicing radiologists from Philadelphia and nearby communities. A series of Tuesday conferences, originally geared toward graduate students, was gradually reoriented toward advanced radiologists, and they gathered at University Hospital to review interesting cases and discuss difficulties.[44] Staff members also worked with the Philadelphia Roentgen Ray Society to organize special seminars and refresher courses, some in conjunction with the American College of Radiology. This commitment to education, and the staff's desire for exposure to inquisitive students as well as to new advances in radiology, kept the creativity, enthusiasm, and competence of the department at a high level.

Growth in the Department Following the War

The department's staff began to expand after the end of World War II; this growth was only partially due to the return of the physicians and technicians who had been serving in the Armed Forces. The residency training program grew considerably during this period, and several of the radiologists who had trained in the mid-1940s remained affiliated with the department following their residencies, so that there were often four or five associates on the staff in addition to eighteen or twenty residents. This growth allowed the physicians to become somewhat more specialized in their responsibilities and allowed the department to expand its areas of investigation and service.

Dr. Pendergrass was gone for several months during 1946, while serving as a Radiation Safety Officer for the postwar atomic bomb tests, but by this time the regular staff had begun to return and there were enough physicians adequately to run the department. Dr. Barden was given full responsibility for the therapy program, the operation in which he had been partially involved with Dr. Pendergrass during the war. With the assistance of Dr. Richard H. Chamberlain, a young physician who completed his

[87]

residency in 1946 and actually ran the treatment program, the operation proceeded smoothly.[45]

The entire world was extremely conscious of radiation exposure following the bombing of Japan, and this attitude presented some difficulties for the department's normal operation. The physicians and physicists had to maintain a sensible approach toward the possibility of hazards and, at the same time, calm patients who were overly concerned about radiation exposure. Careful attention was paid to protective gloves and aprons worn by operators and patients to assure maximum possible safety.

A part-time social worker was first assigned to the department in 1947, and she provided a special contact for therapy patients dealing with practical or emotional problems as a result of their chronic illnesses. Although the department had long been credited with the sensitive care of these patients, the addition of a professional trained to do this type of counseling improved the department's services and relieved the physicians of some of this responsibility.[46]

A new radium room was completed in 1947 and furnished with the most up-to-date equipment for radium therapy.[47] The therapy program was further expanded in the spring of 1948 when a new Brache-Seib superficial therapy machine was installed.[48] Potential difficulties in treatment had arisen in June 1948, when the last Chaoul therapy tube was in use and there was some question as to whether or not replacement tubes existed. Two additional tubes, found in Europe, would serve to alleviate this problem, and the acquisition of the superficial therapy apparatus provided some backup should the Chaoul therapy machine become inoperable.[49] Isotope techniques were also being introduced in the department at this time. Dr. Richard Chamberlain was most closely involved with the expansion of this program.[50]

Improvements were also made to the department's physical plant in 1948, with the beginning of a program to air-condition the entire department. This project was not completed until seven years later, but did provide relief as it was gradually expanded throughout the facility.[51]

Dr. Pendergrass and his associates remained cognizant of the difficulties faced by veterans in the employment market following the war, and at the encouragement of one of his residents he hired a blind veteran to run the department's film processing operation. Minimal design changes were implemented to make the operation compatible with his disability. This proved very successful, setting a precedent which was followed in a number of other departments throughout the nation.[52]

As the decade of the 1940s drew to a close the department was growing steadily, not only because of an increased patient load, but also because new advances in the field of radiology opened a myriad of opportunities for scientists and physicians. The Department of Radiology at University Hospital, always a forerunner in the field, was to maintain its position as the specialty continued to expand.

The Association of Pendergrass Fellows

The Association of Pendergrass Fellows was formed in 1948 by four physicians who had served as residents under Eugene Pendergrass: Fay K. Alexander, George W. Chamberlain, John H. Harris, and Philip J. Hodes, to show their respect, affection, and loyalty for their Chief. In their letter to him, telling of the Association's formation, they further explained that it was to be: ". . . an informal organization which is dedicated to you, to the principles for which you stand, and to friendship."[53]

In the early years the group met annually for a dinner meeting in conjunction with one of the national radiological conferences. The first meeting was in Cincinnati in October, 1949, and the Fellows presented an inscribed silver tray, autographed by all those present, to Dr. Pendergrass. The tray was periodically returned to the engravers for more signatures, and even physicians who were unable to attend the meetings included themselves in this memento.

A magazine, *Grassroots,* was published yearly beginning in 1950. This communication kept track of the various Fellows and their current positions and kept members of the Association up-to-date with the developments in the department at University Hospital. It provided an excellent communications link—former Fellows could find out about current residents and the changes in and additions to the department where they had trained, as well as the activities of their Chief and his colleagues.

At their annual meeting in September, 1951, the members of the Association decided that it would be appropriate for Dr. Pendergrass's portrait to be painted, to be completed in the near future while he still looked as they would remember him. Pendergrass was somewhat reluctant to have the Association pay for the portrait, although he was enthusiastic about its execution, but he eventually agreed to accept the portrait as a gift from the Fellows. It was painted by Roy Spreter, a well-known portrait artist in the Philadelphia and New York areas, and completed in the fall of 1952. The portrait hung in Dr. Pendergrass's home until 1961 when he retired; upon his retirement he gave the portrait to the University and it was hung in the Department of Radiology at the hospital.

In the mid-1950s the Fellows changed the format of their annual meeting and began planning seminar gatherings at various east coast resorts. Early seminars were held at the Greenbriar and at the Homestead, and offered an opportunity for the members of the Association to bring their wives, to play golf or tennis, and to see their old friends. Mornings were spent in seminar sessions with formal presentations by Fellows, offering an opportunity for professional discourse and a tax deduction.

Gatherings of the Association of Pendergrass Fellows continued throughout the decade, and the ranks of the Association grew with each year's class of residents. The establishment of such an organization, inspired by the personal warmth and knowledge of a single physician, explains perhaps more than anything else the calibre of the work in University Hospital's Department of Radiology.

Departmental Operations During the 1950s

As the department's programs and services began to expand during the 1950s, there was a concurrent increase in staff at all levels. However, the growth of the staff did not keep pace with the increase in the patient load due to Dr. Pendergrass's concern about unstable financial conditions, and throughout the mid-1950s he added to the staff only cautiously. A particularly heavy work load was placed on the department's technicians as they assumed responsibility for much of the pre-examination interviewing formerly done by physicians.[54] In addition, some assistance was provided by two technicians' aides who were hired to assist with fluoroscopy.[55]

The radiology installation which opened in the Dulles Building in 1942 had provided ample space for the department's programs at that time, but by the early 1950s the diagnostic and therapeutic facilities were overcrowded and there was a critical shortage of laboratory and research space. The construction of the Thomas S. Gates Memorial Pavilion in the early 1950s provided a major new hospital facility designed for out-patient care, and although the department was not assigned any space in the new building, it was able to plan the expansion of the diagnostic operation into six rooms east of its administrative offices and library, following the relocation of the Obstetrics and Gynecology Clinic. Unfortunately, there was no space available for the simultaneous expansion of the therapeutic and research operations.[56] Long range plans included expanded facilities for these operations in the basements of the Dulles and Gates Pavilions, but these plans were never fully realized.[57]

By 1952 the department had decided to build a large film reading room (subsequently dubbed the "Ball Room") in the new space, as well as to use a portion of it for an out-patient diagnostic clinic which would operate separately from the main radiology facilities. This separate clinical operation served two purposes: one purpose was to isolate patients resident in the hospital from out-patients, and the other was to function as part of the hospital's newly organized Private Diagnostic Clinic. This special clinic, modeled after the Mayo Clinic and partially funded by William H. Donner, opened in 1954 to provide superior diagnostic care by a staff of specialists. This was the first cooperative effort by the hospital's physicians, and it was hoped that Philadelphia corporations would send their employees to the clinic for thorough periodic examinations.[58]

The department formed an independent division under the direction of Dr. Roderick Tondreau, a radiologist who had worked at the Mayo Clinic, to operate this new out-patient facility.[59] His staff included a senior resident, a staff technician, a student technician to work in fluoroscopy, a receptionist, a file clerk, and a darkroom attendant.[60] The new facility was called "Clinic Radiology" or "Out-patient Department" (commonly referred to as the OPD[61]), as opposed to the older diagnostic division, which would be called "Hospital Radiology" or "In-patient Radiology." These titles were somewhat imprecise, however, because the new facility served only two specific groups of out-patients: patients in the Private Diagnostic Clinic and regular clinic out-patients. Private out-patients continued to be examined in the older diagnostic facility, along with hospital in-patients.[62] The new facility was designed to accommodate approximately forty patients each day, thirty-five of whom were clinic out-patients and five of whom were patients in the Private Diagnostic Clinic.[63] There were three fluoroscopic rooms and five radiographic rooms in the separate department; its staff used the "Ball Room" for viewing films with the rest of the staff.[64]

The Private Diagnostic Clinic never achieved substantial success because many of the hospital's physicians still preferred to see all their patients privately rather than to participate in this cooperative program. The Department of Radiology supported the program wholeheartedly, however, and radiological services were donated free of charge in hopes that this might help the Clinic to become self-sufficient.[65] Although it did not attract great numbers of patients for in-depth diagnostic studies, the clinic did provide annual diagnostic examinations for many local corporate executives.[66]

The continued separation of the department into diagnostic and therapeutic divisions contributed to its ongoing efficiency. There was some disruption of general operations in 1953 when the administrative offices were temporarily relocated in the Gates Pavilion during construction, but, as usual, the staff accommodated its work to this added inconvenience.[67] By the mid-1950s the staff was reading clinic films in the afternoon which had been exposed that morning, and was working toward a goal of reporting an entire day's work the same day the films were exposed.[68] Films were checked for technical errors before a patient left the department, preferably before he redressed. This responsibility was assigned to the physician on call, usually a resident; indeed, this procedure was so important that technicians were instructed to ask a senior staff member to read the wet films if the doctor on call was unavailable, rather than delay a patient unnecessarily.[69] Special precautions were taken to insure that the films of private out-patients were properly checked.[70]

Upon completion of the "Ball Room," the department instituted a unique system of film viewing which proved exceedingly successful for both the department's staff and physicians from elsewhere in the hospital. All exposures from hospital ward patients were displayed at the end of each day, and they remained on view throughout the following day. Radiologists and physicians from other departments met at prearranged times every day to jointly review the films of the referring doctors' patients, providing an excellent opportunity for inter-departmental interaction.[71]

Much of the apparatus in the department was purchased in the early 1940s during the move into the new facility, and it had seen hard use during more than ten years of service. Throughout the 1950s purchases were made to upgrade the quality of the apparatus, and, even more importantly, to provide more up-to-date equipment. In 1951 the department purchased two new two-tube radiographic and fluoroscopic units,[72] and a year later a Franklin Angiograph was added to the diagnostic equipment. This piece was designed by Dr. Richard Chamberlain at the University of Pennsylvania, Dr. Edward Chamberlain at Temple University, and Bill Hogan, a local manufacturer of radiologic equipment, and was only the second such piece built (the first was at Temple). It was constructed with two tubes at right angles and could take right angle films simultaneously, as well as stereoscopic films at one-half second intervals. The apparatus, used for procedures requiring serial films, was especially valuable for viewing the heart and vessels of the head, chest, and abdomen.[73] Additional pieces of apparatus were purchased to increase the capabilities for body section tomography, and cinefluorographic equipment was also introduced.[74] In the late 1950s an X-O-Mat mechanical film processing system was installed; it was considerably more efficient and saved a great deal of time, but used ten times more chemicals than earlier equipment had.[75]

The therapy division was particularly interested in the possibilities for supervoltage therapy, but extensive work was delayed until the construction of a new facility toward the end of the decade. Meanwhile, staff members designed and constructed a rotation therapy device, funded by the State Cancer Commission,[76] and added a therapy unit to treat certain forms of deep-seated malignancy.[77] In 1955 a twenty-five milligram radium cell was donated to the department by Frank Hartman.[78]

In 1950 a Physics Committee was established to consider the long range importance of physics in the department's programs. Composed of Drs. Pendergrass, Warren, Chamberlain, Hodes, Hale, and the staff physician at Jeanes Hospital, this group had many responsibilities: analyzing equipment, measuring instruments, assuring the safety of various protective devices in use, developing new apparatus for diagnosis and therapy, and supervising the electronics laboratory.[79]

[93]

Renovation of the reception and waiting areas was completed in the mid-1950s to redirect traffic flow and to modify operations to allow for the separate out-patient facility,[80] and through the generosity of a friend the air-conditioning of the department was completed in 1955. All private patients continued to be examined in the older facility, and for some procedures there were different examination rooms for private and ward patients. There had been a separate entrance for private patients since 1942, and in 1956 a hostess was hired to expedite their examinations and to make their visits as pleasant as possible.[81]

The department's income varied markedly during these years, and there was a continuous problem of nonpayment; in many cases the patients were never even billed. The greatest losses arose from patients examined during the evening and weekend hours, when the regular clerical and administrative staff was not working, and at one point in 1958 the department estimated that only twenty-five percent of the potential clinic income was being collected.[82]

There were additional financial problems because therapy patients were rated by the hospital's billing service, and the calculations made determining their ability to pay were often too low. Many patients were able and willing to pay more than the amount stated for their treatment, but felt that they had been placed in an awkward position by the hospital's billing office.[83] During the summer of 1954 the department changed its therapy billing procedure, however, and thereafter patients were charged for the actual expenses incurred by the department in the course of their treatment. This system worked well, and substantially increased the income received for therapy.[84]

The department usually charged a flat fee for ward examinations, regardless of the number of exposures taken or the degree of difficulty of the procedure.[85] The reimbursement scale for ward patients was graduated, however, dividing them into categories of "full-paid," "part-pay," and "no-pay,"[86] further reducing the amount of the flat fee. Late in the 1950s the department changed its diagnostic rate structure, and began charging ward patients for work actually done. This system financed the true costs of this division's operation.

Administrative, technical, and financial procedures became more involved during the 1950s as the department expanded its services and facilities and saw an ever increasing patient load; nevertheless, superior service for patients continued to be the goal of the entire staff and every effort was made to operate the department in the most efficient and comprehensive manner possible.

Research Programs During the 1950s

The department's staff members carried on a wide variety of research investigations during the decade, which involved the evolution of new techniques, the analysis of clinical data, and the design and construction of new types of apparatus. Work with radioisotopes was just beginning, and this specialization supplemented the established research program in diagnostic and therapeutic radiology.

The explosion of atomic bombs over Japan had generated enormous concern about the effects of radiation exposure, and some staff members pursued the investigation of the biological effects of radiation exposure and their control. This project was begun initially to analyze the impact of radiation on animal life, but was eventually expanded to analyze the effects on humans as well.[87] Much of the research was sponsored by the Army, and also focused on methods of protection from the effects of radiation.[88]

Staff members also worked on the application of television principles to fluoroscopy, in an effort to amplify the fluoroscopic image and thereby improve its quality and reliability. James S. Picker of the Picker X-ray Corporation provided funding for a portion of this research because of his dual interest in improving the fluoroscopic image and in supporting the Department of Radiology at Pennsylvania;[89] the department and the company had worked in close association ever since Dr. Pancoast's time.[90] This project was carried on in the basement laboratory area with the research in both radiation physics and radioisotopes, and resulted in the construction there of an operational unit. By 1954 the apparatus was ready for clinical use, and appropriate patients were taken downstairs to utilize this improved diagnostic apparatus.[91]

Joint research with the Departments of Medicine and Surgery sought to identify forms of cardiovascular disease which were particularly amenable to surgical relief. The success of this research, the early stages of angiography, was due in large part to the apparatus designed by members of the Department of Radiology. Departmental interest in cranial problems prompted a long-

[95]

range analysis which proved especially helpful to the hospital's neurologists and neurosurgeons. Additional diagnostic research involved the reevaluation of the chest roentgenographic routine, and an intensive analysis of procedural and diagnostic fundamentals brought about some substantial changes in both technique and film interpretation.[92]

Analysis of dosage patterns in the treatment of cancer of the cervix was carried on in cooperation with the Department of Gynecology. The close interaction with this department, which began in the late 1940s, directly involved the radiologists in planning therapy programs for gynecology patients, and served to expose physicians in both specialities to new developments in the other field. Additional therapeutic research included a more careful analysis of the measurements used in radiation therapy application.[93]

Research in radiobiology, initiated as part of the isotope program, was expanded considerably in 1958, when a grant from the Fels Fund enabled Dr. Mortimer Mendelsohn to join the department's staff.[94] He concentrated on the utilization of radiational techniques for the investigation of problems in cell biology. The resultant interaction with the scientific research community helped to maintain the department's reputation as a cooperative staff in both the medical and scientific communities, and as one interested in any developments which related to the use of radiation.[95]

The wide scope of the department's research efforts at this time, in addition to an ever-increasing patient load, provided evidence of the staff's deep commitment to the field of radiology. Each physician, from the Chief to the newest resident, was enthusiastically encouraged to pursue his particular interests, and the result was an extensive research program: "It may be stated with just pride that there are few departments in this country, excluding those that are Federal or State owned, where more fundamental research is being done."[96]

Early Work with Radioisotopes

Richard H. Chamberlain began to work with radioisotopes in the department in 1947, and in 1950 the old radium room was converted to laboratory space for this work. A research project gradually developed, investigating the potential uses of isotopes for both diagnostic and therapeutic work, and these new techniques were eventually incorporated into the department's procedures. Chamberlain had assistance from other interested individuals, including the staff physicists, a student physicist, a health physicist, a Fellow, and a technician.[97]

The laboratory space was extremely crowded, but even under such adverse conditions an amazing amount of clinical and research work was accomplished. A therapy program was initiated in 1951 to treat cancer of the thyroid with radioactive iodine, and radioactive colloidal gold was used therapeutically in the treatment of peritoneal and pleural metastasis. Although these treatments were not cures, the new therapeutic programs utilizing radioactive materials offered considerable hope for the future. Radioactive elements were used diagnostically in tracer studies to analyze diseases and the function of internal systems. Staff members also spent time developing new instruments to safely handle and measure activated elements.[98]

Despite consistently difficult working conditions, the scope of work continued to expand. In 1952 clinical work with radio-isotopes included the treatment of severe cardiac disease, as well as treatment for malignant diseases and hyperthyroidism. New diagnostic scanning devices were utilized, and instruments were designed to further minimize the dangers of handling radioactive materials.[99]

In 1953 the hospital's Board of Managers agreed to provide 3,000 square feet of space, in the basement of the Dulles Building under the department's therapy area, for the construction of the Research Radiology Section. Construction was financed by a gift from the Mary Hamilton Kuhn Gordon Cancer Research Fund. The space was equipped with a high level laboratory for radioactive isotope work, electrical and machine shops, physics office space, and a conference room.[100] This space facilitated further expansion of this research throughout the decade.

The Beginning of Work in Nuclear Medicine

David A. Kuhl, a medical student who had studied physics at Temple University as an undergraduate, began to do research in nuclear medicine as soon as he arrived at Pennsylvania in 1951.

Kuhl originally worked in the Physics Research Laboratory, located in the medical school, and his projects complemented the main research in the Department of Radiology. He eventually moved to the Dulles Buidling, into a small room in the middle of the Obstetrics and Gynecology Clinic on the ground floor. In 1953 he moved again, to a convenient location near the electrical and machine shops, when additional space was acquired by the Department of Radiology in the basement of the Dulles Building.[101]

In 1951, while a first year medical student, Kuhl designed his first scanner. Utilizing this scanner and a scintillation detector, he was able to determine radioisotope distribution in the body. The scanner was located in the Physics Laboratory in a corner of the basement of the Dulles Building, to which patients were brought for diagnostic examinations.[102] Kuhl continued to work on the problem of creating images of radioisotope distribution while in medical school, with some financial support from John Hale's grant.[103] In 1955 Kuhl designed and constructed the first photo-recording system to produce a grey-shade record of the radio-isotope deposits in the body viewed by the scanner. This system incorporated a motor-driven detector which moved back and forth across the body of the patient, and used light to create images on film corresponding to the deposits of radioisotopes in different parts of the body.

David Kuhl served his internship at University Hospital from 1955 to 1956, and during that time continued to do work in nuclear medicine in the Department of Radiology. He remained at the hospital for several weeks following his internship before entering the military service, and during that time he continued to see patients. All throughout his medical studies and internship, in fact, he had conducted all the scans on patients himself.

Kuhl returned to the Department of Radiology in the fall of 1958, to serve a regular residency in radiology. His experience and reputation in nuclear medicine had increased considerably during the two years that he was head of the Radioisotope Laboratory at Portsmouth Naval Hospital. When he returned to University Hospital he obtained a grant to support his research. He followed the normal residency program and continued his research work in his spare time. While still a resident he taught courses twice a year in Bethesda.

During 1958 and 1959 David Kuhl and his associates developed the principles of body section tomography in nucleotide scanning, the forerunners of the principles of the EMI Scanner. These early advances in radionucleotide-computed tomography brought about a major breakthrough in nuclear medicine, indicative of the incredibly important work Kuhl was doing while still a resident in the department.

David Kuhl remained in the department following the completion of his residency, and in the early 1960s the division of Nuclear Medicine was formally recognized within the Department of Radiology. Kuhl's contributions to the department's program were recognized as he emerged as one of the most important pioneers in the field of nuclear medicine.[104]

Interaction in the Hospital Community

Joint research and clinical projects with other departments had long been a tradition in the Department of Radiology, but by the 1950s questions arose concerning day-to-day interactions with other departments in the hospital. Radiology's position was somewhat unique, since it provided service for almost every department, and since its operation directly influenced work throughout the hospital. This placed considerable outside pressure on the staff.

Particular difficulties arose when staff members from other departments requested information immediately upon the completion of an examination, before the radiology staff had had time to process and interpret the films. An ever increasing patient load, a growing number of Fellows, and an expanded curriculum for undergraduate medical students placed heavy demands on staff time. The demands of physicians from other departments for an immediate diagnosis of their patients' exposures caused considerably more confusion and inefficiency.

Requests from members of the surgical staff were particularly frequent during 1950 and they prompted Dr. Hodes, then head of the diagnostic division, to seriously consider the department's purpose: was the department, as a department of radiology within a hospital, intended to function as a diagnostic-clinic department, and would it therefore provide immediate service but disrupt the normal organization of the work flow and teaching program? Or, could the department function more independently, maintaining the same autonomy of operation as did others, such as surgery and gynecology? Hodes urged a commitment to cooperative independency, and concluded a memorandum to Dr. Pendergrass in 1950:

No one realizes better than I that ours is a Department dedicated to "service." This is your order to us and it is what all of us are trying to do. But somewhere, "limitless sservice" must stop if the best interests of our Department are to be served. Unless we are prepared to make radical changes and go to considerable expense, we just cannot go on giving this "limitless service."[105]

The specialty of radiology was undergoing introspection everywhere during the 1950s as radiologists considered their role in the expansion into nuclear medicine and the introduction of new procedures, such as angiography, previously considered to be the absolute domain of the surgeon. Members of the Department of Radiology at University Hospital were particularly concerned with these questions.[106]

Radiologists were also concerned about the acceptance of radiology as a medical specialty, rather than a hospital service, by persons outside of the medical profession. The Blue Shield insurance system, for example, would cover the expenses of therapeutic work for a patient treated by a gynecologist or surgeon, but not for a patient treated by a radiologist.[107] This policy generated considerable concern, not only because it placed severe hardships on chronically ill patients, but also because it created difficulties in public relations. Because the department had been treating patients since 1903, the inequities seemed particularly blatant.

Hospital physicians also relied on radiology staff members to participate in other hospital operations, including taking exposures in the operating room. Once this procedure was in progress the surgeon often assumed control, however, and it was difficult for the radiologist, usually a Fellow from the department, to assert his role as a specialist.[108] Such difficulties were, quite obviously, difficult to resolve.

Because Dr. Pendergrass operated the department independently from the hospital, paying the institution on a predetermined sum to cover rent and maintenance, the question of relocating and financing the department's physical expansion was a difficult one. When plans for the Donner Center for Radiology were under consideration in the mid-1950s, additional problems arose between the hospital and the department regarding the division of income received from services in the new building.

Throughout these years, however, the hospital realized the tremendous impact of the Department of Radiology upon the entire institution, and efforts were made to devise mutually acceptable arrangements with consideration given to maintenance of departmental autonomy. Dr. Pendergrass encouraged his staff to try to develop better relations with the hospital administration, in the hope that this would increase the hospital's interest in the department's finances and make it more willing to share some of the expenses.[109]

Teaching Program for Physicians During the 1950s

The expansion of the fellowship program, begun after World War II, continued during the 1950s; in the year 1950 there were twenty-one fellows with plans for even more in the future. The length of the program varied: it was lengthened to four years after the Second World War, shortened to three years from the Korean War into the mid-1950s, and later expanded to four years again. Residents continued to rotate through the Departments of Surgery, Pathology, and Gynecology, and some spent time working at other institutions in or near Philadelphia. They were encouraged to pursue original research as well as to analyze clinical studies, and the staff made every attempt to give each resident a project on which he could work during the years he was in the department.[110] A number of papers were published as a result of this research.[111]

A portion of the rotation through the Department of Surgery was spent in the operating room, providing X-ray coverage. The resident was responsible for the execution of all radiographic procedures during the operation, and he decided the scope of the examination.[112] Residents working in pathology were responsible for organizing cases to be sent to the Armed Forces Institute of Pathology, and throughout the years the department made many contributions to the Institute.[113] The rotation through the Department of Gynecology was closely allied to their specialized cancer treatment program, and offered an unusual opportunity for residents interested in therapy to see its implementation in another department.

[101]

Reciprocal arrangements with Chestnut Hill and Pennsylvania Hospitals enabled Fellows to spend time working in departments which were smaller and more personalized than the one at University Hospital. The radiologist at Jeanes Hospital, a former Fellow under Dr. Pendergrass, encouraged students to rotate there as well. Dr. Pendergrass was also enthusiastic about the opportunities for residents to receive exposure to nonhospital radiology, and was pleased when he was asked to establish a diagnostic facility for the Pennsylvania Manufacturer's Insurance Company. This company, located in center city Philadelphia, equipped a small facility to examine policyholders who had suffered injuries, and a Fellow and a technician from the department ran this operation. This affiliation was structured as a fellowship appointment, as were the trainee positions with the American Cancer Society and the Heublein and DuPont fellowships, and the resident received financial support for his work. The physicians working at Jeanes Hospital during this time were also given small honoraria.[114]

Financing for the continued expansion of the residency training program was substantially aided by a number of trainee positions and fellowships from local and national cancer organizations, industry, and individuals. Many physicians were taken on as residents in their first year or two in the department, and as Fellows in subsequent years; the title change reflected their support from an outside funding source and their individual research projects. Without this outside support the department would have been much more restricted in the scope of its training program.

Pendergrass encouraged Fellows to make clinical visits to other institutions throughout the nation, in addition to their regular hospital rotations. Residents would often go to Massachusetts General Hospital, Columbia University, or the University of Minnesota, and this was thought to be particularly valuable because they were able to compare several superior radiological operations. The Fellows would relate important new developments in radiology which they had observed elsewhere to the staff at University Hospital upon their return.[115]

A great deal of a Fellow's instruction was presented informally, particularly at the many weekly conferences held by the department. Some of these conferences emphasized special subdivisions within the specialty, while others brought together physicians from all over the city to discuss their interesting cases. Many of these conferences focused on diagnostic radiology, but the staff made certain that the residents serving rotations in therapy had an opportunity to attend a variety of conferences while on this rotation as well.[116] In the mid-1950s the department initiated an especially important weekly conference on radiotherapeutics, bringing together physicists, radiobiologists, and radiologists to discuss both the clinical and the theoretical aspects of radiation therapy. Its reputation grew quickly, and the weekly meetings received favorable comment throughout the United States.[117] The conferences reemphasized the department's concern for continuing medical education, and its willingness to serve the entire medical community.

The diagnostic training for Fellows centered on practical experience, and residents were given responsibility for reading films shortly after their initial instruction. These films were usually from clinic and hospital ward patients, and the Fellows' diagnoses were later double-checked by members of the senior staff. This approach extended the resident's responsibility, because he was forced to make his own analysis of the films, without any immediate feedback, and only later learned whether or not the experienced staff agreed with his diagnosis.[118]

Residents were encouraged to work with Dr. Chamberlain and his research with radioisotopes in the basement, and to apply for special training in this field if they were interested.[119] Exposure to the scanning and related nuclear medicine procedures also came while on the job.[120] A new teaching file system was introduced in 1954, and this resource proved helpful for Fellows, staff, and medical students.[121]

There were some changes in the department's operation during the Korean War, and as had been the case during prior conflicts, the staff was involved in programs to train medical personnel in radiology. In most cases, however, some emphasis on military medicine was added to the normal curriculum, rather than developing an entirely separate program for members of the Armed Forces.[122]

The University and the Department of Radiology tried very hard to protect their students from the military draft so that there would be a continuous supply of specialists in the field; nonetheless, a number of the department's residents left in the middle of their training to serve in the military, and returned after their tours of duty to complete their work in radiology. Some accelerated their training, enabling them to complete the program before they left the department, and the entire program was shortened from four years to three years during this time.[123]

Graduate instruction in the department was not limited solely to the fellowship program. In 1951 the department cosponsored an interdisciplinary course leading to a Ph.D., combining work with other departments from the School of Medicine and the Departments of Physics, Mathematics, and Engineering. Beginning in 1958, when Mortimer Mendelsohn joined the staff, special projects were initiated in radiobiology, including research in cell biology.[124]

In addition to their own instruction, Fellows were given teaching responsibilities for the interns passing through the department and for students in the School of Medicine. The responsibilities regarding the interns were the same for each member of the staff: they were assigned an individual intern, escorted him around the department, explained the various programs, and generally acted in the capacity of instructor for the duration of the intern's short stay.[125] The Fellows' more extensive responsibility as educators, however, was toward undergraduate medical students. Changes in the school curriculum in the early 1950s considerably expanded the number of courses offered in radiology, and residents taught the fundamentals of radiology during the first and second years in order to properly prepare medical students for electives in their third and fourth years.

Some Fellows were assigned full-time to the Departments of Anatomy and Physiology, and worked closely with first year students in these two departments. In anatomy the resident provided some assistance in dissection, but was most responsible for teaching roentgen anatomy; in physiology he gave fluoroscopic demonstrations of the pulmonary, cardiovascular, and intestinal systems. During the second year of instruction residents worked in pathology, helping in the laboratory area, performing autopsies, and demonstrating the roentgen manifestations of disease. Considerable time was also spent correlating pathological conditions with their roentgenographic manifestations. In addition, the second year included some time spent in didactic lectures, with some instruction in diagnostic radiology.

This preparation in radiology provided a suitable background for students to come to the department for electives during their third year, and four students rotated through the department every two-and-a-half weeks, spending full days there. The fourth year of instruction concentrated on clinico-radiological conferences, emphasizing cancer diagnosis and treatment. Besides these formal courses of instruction, a number of interested students spent summers as externs in the department as well, usually between their third and fourth years of medical school.[126]

The overall expansion in the Department of Radiology during the 1950s provided more diversified educational programs on all levels than ever before, and greater opportunities for Fellows to work with senior staff members in a wide variety of special research projects. Following the Korean War, the length of the residency was again extended to four years to provide sufficient time for instruction in radiation therapy; quotas for time in various subdivisions of the specialty were now dictated by outside groups, especially the American Medical Association and the American College of Radiology, as much as by the wishes of the department's staff. With a variety of opportunities for specialization and outside work, study in the department offered the Fellow an excellent combination of general diagnostic and therapeutic radiology and exposure to the specialities within the field.

Educational Programs in the School
for X-Ray Technicians

The School for X-ray Technicians experienced difficulties during the Second World War, but continued in operation. By the early 1950s its structure had evolved into a series of classroom courses and preceptorial instruction involving the entire department. Classwork received priority in the students' schedule, however, and the department's staff did its best to enable students to reach their classes promptly.[127]

The department's concern for quality education was just as evident in its approach to the instruction of technicians as it was in the residency training program. Students were taught the fundamentals of X-ray technology in their classes, and were later exposed to a variety of X-ray techniques by working with physicians and experienced technicians.

First year students in the two year curriculum were rotated throughout the various divisions of the department in order fully to acquaint them with the department's operation, and changed services every two weeks.[128] In addition to their learning experiences, student technicians provided backup for the permanent staff, and two student technicians, as well as two Fellows, were always assigned to therapy to provide adequate coverage.[129]

The department's staff was concerned that the student technicians learn more than the mere fundamentals of X-ray technology while in the department, and care was taken to see that they were given responsibility as soon as they were qualified to work independently. This opportunity to act independently helped the sagging morale of the students in the program in the early 1950s, and made them feel as though they were really part of the department. The supportive and encouraging attitude adopted by staff members bolstered the students' confidence and enabled them to complete the program with a degree of maturity equal to their technical competence.[130] The program continued successfully during the 1950s and rounded out the scope of training offered by the department.

The William H. Donner Center for Radiology

Expansion into the Out-patient Department somewhat alleviated the severe overcrowding of diagnostic facilities, but there was still a shortage of space which inhibited the expansion of specialized diagnostic and therapeutic procedures and advances in the research in isotopes and radiobiology. Dr. Chamberlain drew up specifications for an Isotope and Radiobiology Wing in 1952, to be added to the present hospital building, and although an estimate was obtained, funding for this project never materialized.

The department eventually developed plans for a more comprehensive expansion program, incorporating projects in supervoltage roentgenology and fluoroscopic amplification, in addition to the work in isotopes and radiobiology, and made a formal presentation to the Donner Foundation in September, 1954. The proposal stressed the quality of the department's personnel, and emphasized the fact that their full potential could be realized only if they had adequate facilities and opportunities. William H. Donner had always demonstrated a preference for investing his money in people rather than in bricks and mortar, and the tone of the appeal, therefore, highlighted these aspects:

These men, with training in several disciplines, are functioning as a team that has already attracted attention and has received major support from several sources. An excellent job has been done with limited facilities and equipment. Members of the Department have the interest and desire to record still greater progress in their chosen specialty—but this can be realized only if additional space and tools are available to them.[131]

Mr. Donner had died the year before, but the foundation was still very interested in the department's work, and in late September its Board approved a gift of $750,000: $500,000 for the construction of a building adjoining the hospital, and the balance to begin a permanent endowment whose income would cover some of the operating expenses. The new building was to be called the William H. Donner Center for Radiology. The United States Public Health Service also provided $180,000 in matching funds toward the construction of research facilities in the Center.[132]

The construction of a new facility was especially exciting, because it enabled the department to develop extensive plans for supervoltage roentgenology procedures. Supervoltage therapy was particularly valuable in the treatment of carcinoma of the esophagus, bladder, cervix, and head and neck.[133] The Donner Foundation donated a two-million-electron-volt Van de Graaff generator for therapy in the new Center, and a one-million-electron-volt diagnostic research machine was obtained through a United States Public Health Service grant.[134] The department was able to accept the latter piece specifically because it would have an acceptable research facility in which to house it.

Supervoltage roentgenology had long been of interest to William Donner; years earlier, when Eugene Pendergrass first asked for money to purchase such equipment, Mr. Donner had been amazed to learn how expensive it was. The men met with the president of the High Voltage Engineering Corporation, one firm manufacturing such equipment, and learned that each piece was practically handmade. He assured them, however, that production in quantity would be considerably less expensive, so Mr. Donner decided to donate a dozen supervoltage units to hospitals around the United States. With Dr. Pendergrass's help he identified institutions which were centrally located, and developed cooperative arrangements whereby physicians from all over a region were able to use the equipment installed in a single location.[135] It was particularly fitting, therefore, that supervoltage roentgenology tied in so closely with the new Donner Center.

As soon as the Donner Foundation approved the gift, plans for the building were initiated and the department's staff was invited to make suggestions for its design.[136] There were several revisions of the plans, however, and they were not finally approved by the foundation until December, 1955. Dr. Richard Chamberlain was deeply involved in the design of the building, partially due to his earlier design for the proposed isotope and radiobiology wing. Construction bids for the building were considerably higher than the $500,000 originally allocated by the foundation, and although the board agreed to increase the construction budget to $600,000, the design plans were also necessarily simplified. Construction of the building began on September 28, 1956, nearly two years after announcement of the gift.

Construction of the Donner Center created some administrative difficulties between the department, the University, and the hospital, because the gift was actually made to the University. The University administration wanted input in the delineation of specific plans for the Center's organization, operation, and research program, while the hospital was particularly concerned that it would lose therapy income, since treatments would be given in a University facility, rather than a hospital building.

In the past the hospital had received the income from clinic and ward patients receiving treatment or undergoing examinations, and the department had received income from private patients, but with an expansion of services in the new building to include an increasing number of radioisotope procedures for both diagnosis and therapy, the allocation of income from these procedures was in question. After much discussion and consultation, it was decided that the hospital would receive all patient income except that from new procedures, and that the income generated by these new procedures would be returned to the Center, to create an ongoing research fund. The University agreed to pay the hospital for the Center's housekeeping costs, relieving the department of that financial burden.

The Department of Radiology did not receive additional direct income from the Donner Center, and it actually lost some sources of income, since the money from private patients, formerly paid to the department, now went to the hospital if the work was carried out in the Donner Center. Staff time was devoted to work in the Center without reimbursement from the hospital or University. In general, though, the establishment of the Center provided many opportunities for expansion of staff activities, and the department still received considerable outside funding to cover the costs of special research projects going on in the Center. The hospital was often operating at a deficit at this time, and the department's agreement to give to the hospital all income from established procedures executed in the Donner Center was one way of easing some of the hospital's financial burdens.

The staff of the department began to move into the new building in late December, 1957, and the Donner Center was formally dedicated and opened to the public on February 28, 1958.[137] The completion of this facility provided, for the first time, expanded space for research in radioisotopes and radiobiology as well as room to house large pieces of therapy equipment.[138]

National Prominence

Besides their extensive clinical, teaching, and research activities at the hospital and University, staff members of the Department of Radiology were active participants in national radiological and medical societies. Some served as officers or on important policy and planning committees, while others were invited to present annual orations and lectures sponsored each year by various organizations. These activities and awards were but one more indication of the calibre of the department's staff, and the recognition given it at the national level.

Eugene Pendergrass's outside activities during the 1950s were especially noteworthy in view of his responsibilities as Chief and his commitment to the ongoing expansion of the department's program. He served as President of the Radiological Society of North America during 1954, as a delegate to the Section on Radiology of the American Medical Association beginning in 1957, and as President of the American Cancer Society from 1958 to 1959. He was invited to give the Tenth Annual Pancoast Lecture to the Philadelphia Roentgen Ray Society in 1950, and the Caldwell Lecture to the American Roentgen Ray Society in 1957. He received the Gold Medal of the American College of Radiology in 1956, and the Gold Medal of the Radiological Society of North America in 1957.

The activities of the rest of the staff followed this example of excellence: members of the Department of Radiology continually brought honor to their department, University, and hospital. The scope of their commitment, supported by their outstanding capabilities, ensured the success and prestige of the entire operation.

Eugene Percival Pendergrass— Emeritus Professor and Chief

After more than forty years of service at Pennsylvania, Eugene P. Pendergrass retired in 1961. He was succeeded as Chairman by Richard Hall Chamberlain, his long-time associate and Chief of the department's radiotherapy program.[139] Dr. Pendergrass turned over the entire operation to Dr. Chamberlain, but continued to practice medicine. The Department of Radiology at Jeanes Hospital needed additional staffing to enable Dr. Edwin L. Lame, a former Pendergrass Fellow, to accept an administrative position at Pennsylvania, so Pendergrass spent the first two years of his "retirement" working there. A close associate on the staff at Jeanes was Dr. Nathan Salner, another former Fellow.[140] From 1962 to 1966 Dr. Pendergrass served as Director of the Bicentennial Observance of the School of Medicine.

Dr. Pendergrass continued to serve as a consultant, particularly on silicosis and related diseases, but he was also interested in new developments in radiology. He was named the first Matthew J. Wilson Professor of Research Radiology, and held that position from 1964 to 1966. In later years he remained active in various radiological and medical societies, as well as on University committees, and served as a trustee of the Presbyterian-University of Pennsylvania Medical Center and as a consultant to the Department of Radiology of the Japan National Institute of Health.

The Association of Pendergrass Fellows continued to meet every few years: in 1965 they held a dinner at the Faculty Club in honor of Dr. and Mrs. Pendergrass and in 1970, on his seventy-fifth birthday, a gala celebration at The Barclay Hotel included the Associates and several distinguished European physicians.[141] Dr. Pendergrass spent time in his hospital office daily until the fall of 1978, and welcomed the opportunity to meet with old patients and friends as well as old and new staff members.

NOTES

1. Hospital of the University of Pennsylvania, *Annual Report of the Board of Managers* (31 May 1941), p. 68.

2. Hospital of the University of Pennsylvania, *Annual Report of the Board of Managers* (31 May 1946), p. 56.

3. Eugene P. Pendergrass, Personal Interview, 17 June 1976.

4. Hospital of the University of Pennsylvania, *Annual Report of the Board of Managers* (31 May 1939), p. 70; Hospital of the University of Pennsylvania, *Annual Report of the Board of Managers* (31 May 1940), p. 69.

5. Hospital of the University of Pennsylvania, *Annual Report,* 1941, p. 67.

6. Department of Radiology, Hospital of the University of Pennsylvania, "Interne's Register, Comments of James D. Maxwell" (1941), p. 109.

7. *Ibid.,* "Comments of Charles D. Merckel" (1941), p. 108.

8. *Ibid.,* "Comments of Joseph H. Hafhenschiel" (1941), p. 117.

9. Eugene P. Pendergrass and Robert P. Barden, "Radiological Service Advanced by Design," *Modern Hospital* 60, No. 6 (1943): 68–70.

10. Hospital of the University of Pennsylvania, *Annual Report,* 1941, p. 67.

11. Pendergrass, Personal Interview, 10 August 1976.

12. Eugene P. Pendergrass, "Comments on the Department's Activities," c. 1943.

13. Department of Radiology Staff Physicians, Hospital of the University of Pennsylvania, *Meeting Minutes,* 24 August 1942.

14. *Ibid.,* 28 December 1942.   15. *Ibid.,* 24 August 1942.

16. *Ibid.,* 24 July 1944.   17. *Ibid.,* 22 May 1944.

18. Pendergrass, "Comments." 19. *Ibid.*

20. Department of Radiology, *Minutes,* 28 June 1943.

21. *Ibid.,* 24 July 1943.

22. Hospital of the University of Pennsylvania, *Annual Report,* 1941, p. 68.

23. Pendergrass, "Comments." 24. *Ibid.*

25. Department of Radiology, *Minutes,* May 1945.

26. *Ibid.,* 28 June 1943.   27. Pendergrass, "Comments."

28. *Ibid.*

29. Department of Radiology, *Minutes,* 24 April 1943.

30. *Ibid.,* 28 June 1943.

31. Pendergrass, Personal Interview, 10 August 1976.

32. *Ibid.*

33. Pendergrass, "Comments."

34. Department of Radiology, *Minutes,* 27 October 1947.

35. *Ibid.,* 26 September 1949.   36. *Ibid.,* 27 July 1942.

37. *Ibid.,* 24 April 1943. 38. *Ibid.,* 26 May 1947.

39. *Ibid.,* 24 April 1944.

40. Robert P. Barden, Personal Interview, 16 March 1976.

41. Department of Radiology, *Minutes,* 25 January 1943.

42. *Ibid.,* 28 February 1944.

43. Pendergrass, Personal Interview, 10 August 1976.

44. Department of Radiology, *Minutes,* 25 March 1946.

45. Barden, Personal Interview, 16 March 1976.

46. Department of Radiology, *Minutes,* 26 May 1947.

47. *Ibid.,* 23 December 1947. 48. *Ibid.,* 26 April 1948.

49. *Ibid.,* 26 June 1948. 50. *Ibid.,* 23 December 1947.

51. *Ibid.,* 24 May 1948. 52. *Ibid.,* 28 January 1949.

53. Steering Committee, Pendergrass Associates to Eugene P. Pendergrass, 18 May 1948, Department of Radiology Records and Registers, Pendergrass Associates, Hospital of the University of Pennsylvania, Philadelphia.

54. Department of Radiology, *Minutes,* 27 December 1954.

55. *Ibid.,* 24 May 1954.

56. Hospital of the University of Pennsylvania, *Annual Report of the Board of Managers* (31 May 1952), p. 40.

57. *Grassroots,* Official Organ of the Association of Pendergrass Fellows (1952): 3.

58. Pendergrass, Personal Interview, 10 August 1976; Hospital of the University of Pennsylvania, *Annual Report of the Board of Managers* (31 May 1954), p. 3.

59. *Grassroots* (1954): 9.

60. Department of Radiology, *Minutes,* 18 January 1954.

61. John Hale, Written Comments, Fall 1976.

62. Department of Radiology Staff Technicians and Secretaries, Hospital of the University of Pennsylvania, *Meeting Minutes,* 20 October 1953, 18 February 1954.

63. Department of Radiology, *Minutes,* 18 January 1954.

64. *Grassroots* (1954): 9.

65. Pendergrass, Personal Interview, 17 June 1976.

66. Department of Radiology, *Minutes,* 26 May 1958.

67. Hospital of the University of Pennsylvania, *Annual Report of the Board of Managers* (31 May 1953), p. 38.

68. Philip J. Hodes to Eugene P. Pendergrass, 31 May 1950, Department of Radiology Records and Registers, Miscellaneous Papers, Hospital of the University of Pennsylvania, Philadelphia.

69. Radiology Technicians and Secretaries, *Minutes,* 17 April 1951.

70. Department of Radiology, *Minutes,* 24 January 1955.

71. *Grassroots* (1954): 9.

72. Hospital of the University of Pennsylvania, *Annual Report of the Board of Managers* (31 May 1951), p. 36.

73. Hospital of the University of Pennsylvania, *Annual Report,* 1952, pp. 40–41; *Grassroots* (1952): 2.

74. Hospital of the University of Pennsylvania, *Annual Report,* 1952, pp. 40–41; Hospital of the University of Pennsylvania, *Annual Report of the Board of Managers* (31 May 1961), p. 42; Department of Radiology, *Minutes,* 24 January 1955.

75. Adele K. Friedman, Personal Interview, Spring 1976; Department of Radiology, *Minutes,* 22 October 1958.

76. Hospital of the University of Pennsylvania, *Annual Report,* 1952, p. 40.

77. *Ibid.,* p. 36.

78. Department of Radiology, *Minutes,* 24 October 1955.

79. *Grassroots* (1950): 6.

80. Hospital of the University of Pennsylvania, *Annual Report of the Board of Managers* (31 May 1956), p. 4.

81. Department of Radiology, *Minutes,* 27 February 1956.

82. *Ibid.,* 28 July 1958.

83. Radiology Technicians and Secretaries, *Minutes,* 20 May 1954.

84. *Ibid.,* 28 October 1954.

85. Department of Radiology, *Minutes,* 28 September 1959.

86. *Ibid.,* 20 June 1960.

87. Hospital of the University of Pennsylvania, *Annual Report,* 1951, p. 36.

88. Hospital of the University of Pennsylvania, *Annual Report,* 1952, p. 40.

89. Hospital of the University of Pennsylvania, *Annual Report,* 1951, p. 36.

90. Pendergrass, Personal Interview, 11 August 1976.

91. Department of Radiology, *Minutes,* 26 April 1954.

92. Hospital of the University of Pennsylvania, *Annual Report,* 1952, p. 40.

93. *Ibid.*

94. Department of Radiology, *Minutes,* 28 October 1957.

95. George W. Corner, *Two Centuries of Medicine: A History of the School of Medicine, University of Pennsylvania* (Philadelphia: J. B. Lippincott, 1965).

96. Hospital of the University of Pennsylvania, *Annual Report,* 1952, p. 40.

97. *Grassroots* (1950): 3.

98. Hospital of the University of Pennsylvania, *Annual Report,* 1951, p. 36.

99. Hospital of the University of Pennsylvania, *Annual Report,* 1952, p. 40.

100. Hale, Written Comments, Fall 1976.

101. David E. Kuhl, Personal Interview, 10 March 1976.

102. *Ibid.*

103. Hale, Written Comments, Fall 1976.

104. Kuhl, Personal Interview, 10 March 1976.

105. Hodes to Pendergrass, 31 May 1950.

106. Department of Radiology, *Minutes*, 23 June 1952.

107. *Ibid.*, 26 October 1953.

108. *Ibid.*, 23 May 1955.

109. *Ibid.*, 26 January 1959.

110. *Ibid.*, 24 January 1955.

111. *Grassroots* (1950): 6.

112. Department of Radiology, *Minutes*, 23 May 1955.

113. *Ibid.*, 28 July 1958.

114. Pendergrass, Personal Interview, 11 August 1976.

115. *Ibid.*

116. Department of Radiology, *Minutes*, 27 October 1958.

117. Hospital of the University of Pennsylvania, *Annual Report*, 1953, p. 38.

118. Department of Radiology, *Minutes*, 27 July 1959.

119. *Ibid.*, 27 September 1954.

120. Kuhl, Personal Interview, 10 March 1976.

121. Department of Radiology, *Minutes*, 22 November 1954.

122. *Grassroots* (1951): 1.

123. *Ibid.*

124. Corner, *Medicine.*

125. Department of Radiology, *Minutes*, 25 February 1952.

126. *Grassroots* (1951):2.

127. Radiology Technicians and Secretaries, *Minutes*, 20 October 1953.

128. *Ibid.*, 28 October 1954.

129. *Ibid.*, 21 January 1952.

130. *Ibid.*, 1951.

131. Department of Radiology, Hospital of the University of Pennsylvania, "Proposal to the Donner Foundation, September, 1954," p. 8, Research Files, Donner Center and Foundation, Hospital of the University of Pennsylvania, Philadelphia.

132. *Grassroots* (1957): 26.

133. *Ibid.* (1951): 4.

134. *Ibid.* (1957): 26.

135. Pendergrass, Personal Interview, 17 June 1976.

136. Department of Radiology, *Minutes*, 22 November 1954.

137. Hospital of the University of Pennsylvania, *Annual Report of the Board of Managers* (31 May 1958), p. 3.

138. Department of Radiology, Hospital of the University of Pennsylvania, "Correspondence and Plans Relating to the Donner Center, December 1952 through March 1958," Department Records and Regis-

ters, Donner Center and Foundation, Hospital of the University of Pennsylvania, Philadelphia.

139. Hospital of the University of Pennsylvania, *Annual Report,* 1961 p. 16.

140. Pendergrass, Personal Interview, 11 August 1976.

141. *University of Pennsylvania Medical Center Annual Report 1970–71* (Philadelphia: 1971).

THE CHAMBERLAIN ERA
1960–1975

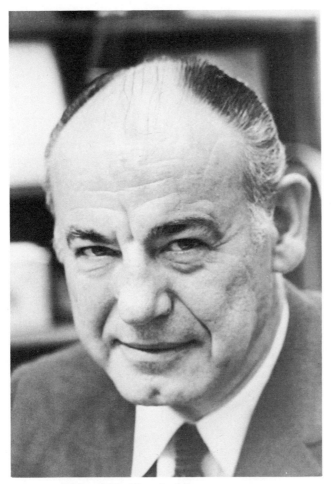

Richard H. Chamberlain, 1961–1975

Richard Hall Chamberlain—
Early Biographical Information

Richard H. Chamberlain was born in Jacksonville, Florida in 1915, and received his Bachelor of Arts Degree in 1934, when only 19 years old, from Centre College in Danville, Kentucky. He taught school for a year in rural Kentucky, then entered the University of Louisville School of Medicine in 1935. Chamberlain completed medical school four years later and following a year-long rotating internship at Louisville City Hospital came east to accept a fellowship in radiology at the Hospital of the University of Pennsylvania.

Dr. Chamberlain spent two years in the residency program, and in 1942 entered active military service as a radiologist in the U.S. Army. He was originally assigned to the 20th General Hospital in India, the unit staffed by University Hospital personnel, but eventually served as Chief of the Radiology Service at the 24th Station Hospital in Persia and Nichols General Hospital in India.[1]

Richard H. Chamberlain returned to the hospital in 1946, and took over the operation of the department's radiotherapy program. He was promoted to the rank of Professor in 1952 and assigned specific duties as Chief of the Therapeutic Division at the same time that Philip J. Hodes was assigned responsibility for the Diagnostic Division.[2] Chamberlain also initiated the department's radioisotope program in the late 1940s, and worked with other associates to design new apparatus for the department.

Departmental Operations Under Chamberlain

Richard H. Chamberlain had his own style and priorities for radiologic service, and it was only natural that there were some changes in the department's operations once he became Chairman. The department also faced new external developments at this time, particularly the increase in specialization within the discipline of radiology and continual changes in its relationship with the hospital.

[119]

Dr. Chamberlain was not especially interested in the administrative operation of the department, so he asked a friend and long-time associate, Dr. Edward M. DeYoung, if he would join the staff as administrator. Dr. DeYoung agreed, and thus became the first physician in the United States to serve as a departmental administrator. He also spent about one-third of his time reading films.[3]

Edward M. DeYoung spent most of his medical career in the U.S. Army and during World War II was stationed at a regular Army hospital across the street from the 20th General Hospital. Philip J. Hodes ran the radiology service at the 20th and held weekly film reading sessions for all the nearby radiologists, so Dr. DeYoung got to know him and other members of the University Hospital staff at this time. After the war he spent a year at University Hospital taking a refresher course in radiation therapy under Richard Chamberlain, during which they became close friends. Although there were only a few familiar faces in the Department of Radiology when Dr. DeYoung returned in 1961, many of his World War II friends still worked elsewhere in the hospital.[4]

Richard H. Chamberlain was interested in the increasing specialization within the discipline of radiology, and most especially the evolution of distinct specialities within diagnostic and therapeutic radiology. A staffing structure indicative of these developments would include a number of specialists with responsibility for a narrow scope of the overall operation and a small staff working under each of them. The importance of such a structure was reinforced as new discoveries and techniques continually increased the amount of knowledge required by a practicing radiologist. Dr. Chamberlain sought to implement such a staffing arrangement in his department, but a tight fiscal position prohibited the addition of a sufficient number of physicians to make this type of operation viable.[5]

The senior staff was small throughout the 1960s. There were only a few diagnostic radiologists, and at the beginning of the decade they were young and fairly inexperienced.[6] None of these physicians had the type of specialized background in which Dr. Chamberlain was particularly interested, so the diagnostic operation functioned without a leader until 1972, when the responsibility was officially delegated to Wallace T. Miller. Chamberlain's appointment of Miller as Chief of Diagnosis was a step back from his philosophical position, but there were still not sufficient funds

[120]

to implement the more specialized structure.[7] The lack of delegation of authority within the diagnostic staff, and its continued small size, were particularly frustrating to its staff members since this part of the department generated a great deal of income each year.[8]

Dr. Chamberlain did not officially delegate authority for the therapy program either, but for several years Dr. Antolin Raventos's seniority enabled him to run the operation with a free hand. The therapy staff remained small, but Dr. Raventos was able to exert considerable influence in the decision making process. Chamberlain was equally supportive of the specialized work being done by David E. Kuhl in nuclear medicine and Mark M. Mishkin in neuroradiology; these physicians worked independently and were actively encouraged to pursue research projects.[9]

At the beginning of the decade operational procedures in the department remained at a *status quo* position: private and ward patients were physically separated in the department, senior staff members performed procedures on private patients and read their films, while residents performed procedures on ward patients and read ward films, which were later checked by senior physicians. Fairly soon, however, the department began to mix private and ward patients, and the department's residents were given increasing responsibility for day-to-day operations. The increased responsibility vested in the residents meant that many patients lost contact with their primary care physician, and the department lost a number of patients due to this nonpersonalized service.[10] The department also provided therapy treatment for patients from Children's Hospital, and departmental residents were responsible for training residents from Children's Hospital in diagnostic procedures.[11]

A tight fiscal situation within the department, and the lack of a strong commitment from the hospital, hindered the acquisition of replacements for standard pieces of apparatus. Much of it had deteriorated from continual usage, and no provisions were made to update the equipment.[12] The department's fluoroscopic apparatus was converted to image-intensified pieces during these years,[13] but some pieces of equipment, such as a pluri-directional unit, were acquired several years after they became standard apparatus elsewhere.[14]

The department was more successful, however, in acquiring specialized or experimental pieces of apparatus. A six-million-electron-volt linear accelerator was dedicated in June, 1965; it was the first such piece in Philadelphia and one of fewer than fifty units nationwide. It was designed to focus the full intensity of its supervoltage X-ray beam in the treatment of cancer.[15] Three years later special magnification apparatus was added to facilitate angiographic procedures.[16]

Richard H. Chamberlain and his associates continued to design and construct apparatus for use in the department, and in 1970 they were able to begin the clinical evaluation of the multiplane, orbital "superfluoroscope" which they had built. This unit, which was absolutely unique, could be used to view a patient from any angle at any space orientation. It was particularly useful to examine the spinal cord, gall bladder, and stomach.[17]

The improvement and modernization of clinical facilities was an ongoing, though low-key, activity, and in 1973 plans were finalized to add a multidirectional tomographic unit and ultrasound capabilities to the department's diagnostic operation.[18] In December, 1974 the department received its EMI Scanner, a unit based on many of the principles developed by David E. Kuhl in his nuclear medicine research and first developed in England three-and-one-half years earlier. This apparatus was so sophisticated, and designed to record so many different views nearly simultaneously, that the equations collected as data were solved by a computer to create the image which was later interpreted by the radiologist.[19]

The department's long standing commitment to radiological research was greatly enhanced in 1961, when the announcement was formally made of the Matthew J. Wilson Professorship in Research Radiology. The endowed chair, named for a distinguished Philadelphia physician and civic leader, was made possible by a series of gifts from his children, Matthew J. Wilson, Jr. and Mrs. Fred C. Newcombe. The young Wilson had been a patient of Dr. Pendergrass's some twenty-five years earlier, and was so impressed with the department that he had sent the Chairman a generous contribution. Additional gifts from him and his sister were equally substantial, and Dr. Pendergrass felt obligated to ask for their input on the use of this money. Both were pleased at the suggestion of an endowed chair in memory of their father, and once their gifts exceeded the sum of $500,000 an announcement was officially made. Most appropriately, Eugene P. Pendergrass was the first physician appointed to hold this chair.[20]

Staff members continued to work on a variety of research projects during these years. Diagnostic research included such diverse topics as urethral tumors, retroperitoneal fibrosis, and renal trauma, while a study of pericardial effusions compared the values of ultrasound, radioisotope scanning, and cinefluorographic methods. There was also ongoing investigation of the merits of conventional *versus* high kilovoltage chest techniques.[21] A cooperative research program was begun in the early 1970s with the School of Veterinary Medicine in its excellent research facilities, which enabled residents and staff members to improve their clinical technique for procedures such as catheterization in angiography.[22] At the Veterans Administration Hospital, joint research in diagnostic radiology and nuclear medicine centered on cardiac visualization.[23]

Research projects in therapeutic radiology included the application of computers to calculate radiation dosage for external beam therapy machines and the interstitial and intracavity implants of radioactive materials. Work continued with the application of high LET radiation to treat malignant disease. Dr. James Brennan, holder of the department's endowed chair in Research Radiology, continued his work with the therapeutic potential of fast neutron treatment. The successful development of a neutron generator target, after considerable work, enabled him and his colleagues to consider the construction of a practical clinical unit to use in the treatment of human cancer.[24]

Dr. Mortimer Mendelsohn continued his research in radiobiology. Specific projects undertaken by him and his associates included the investigation of better methods to create images of human chromosomes, the study of tumor kinetics, and the measurement of cell death.[25] Prior to his departure for California in the fall of 1972, he and his colleagues were able to use their techniques for image analysis to measure the DNA content of human chromosome sets with sufficient resolution to identify twenty chromosome types, and in some cases to isolate individual chromosomes rather than homologous pairs.[26]

The department continued to use the control room, where residents checked films prior to a patient's departure, through 1975, although by 1970 the patient load was too great for it to operate effectively because there were too many films to keep organized.[27] A continued increase in the patient load also precipitated some modifications of the department's physical layout: examination rooms for brief procedures were relocated near the entrance, and more lengthy procedures moved further back in the department.[28] The opening of the Ravdin Courtyard facility in the fall of 1972 provided additional waiting room and office space, facilitating the department's overall operation. At the same time, the introduction of computer technology assisted with the handling of routine appointments and patient data.[29]

Richard H. Chamberlain was able to retain the department's independent status throughout most of his chairmanship, although such a position became increasingly difficult to maintain. There were almost yearly changes in the specific details of his arrangements with the hospital, but he was successful in negotiating a better fee schedule than that under which Dr. Pendergrass had operated.[30] The continuation of departmental autonomy clearly had advantages, but it also minimized the commitment felt by the hospital toward the department's operation, physical plant, and equipment.[31]

In general, the department paid the hospital one-half of all fees collected from in-patients and kept all fees collected from private out-patients. No charge was made by the department for clinic out-patients, and the hospital was supposed to earmark any fees which it collected from these patients for the Radiology Fund. Continued difficulties with insurance reimbursement for radiological procedures (hospital *versus* physicians' services and Blue Cross *versus* Blue Shield), and complications added by the Medicare program, eventually caused the department to turn over the entire collection process to the hospital.[32]

Dr. Chamberlain and the hospital administration agreed to make equal contributions toward equipment purchase, although all apparatus was to become the property of the hospital.[33] This arrangement proved particularly frustrating, however, because the hospital was never willing to contribute more than $50,000 in any given year; Dr. Chamberlain would have willingly contributed three times that much. At this time a budget of $100,000 did not permit the purchase of very much apparatus, and the department was not able to replace much of its standard equipment, or to keep pace with all the advances in radiological technology.[34]

Dr. Chamberlain continued to pay the salaries of the department's technical and support staff during most of his chairmanship, although there was increasing pressure for them to become hospital employees. In later years he was contracted by the hospital to be its "employment agent," and he paid these salaries from a lump sum given him by the hospital. There was also some pressure for the physicians to become hospital employees during the 1960s, but their salaries continued to be paid by the Chairman.[35] Dr. Chamberlain continued the practice of contributing a portion of their salaries to the University to qualify them for its pension and benefit programs. When an individual was included in a University-sponsored funding grant, Dr. Chamberlain had only to pay the difference between the funding and the base salary figure.[36] The department also benefited directly from a number of outside funding sources: the American Cancer Society, the American Medical Association, the Atomic Energy Commission, the National Institutes of Health, the United States Public Health Service, the Picker Foundation, the Fred C. and Charlotte Wilson Newcombe Memorial Trust, and the Matthew J. and Anne C. Wilson Trust Fund.[37]

The staff of the Department of Radiology continued to provide the best service it could throughout these years. There were some frustrations: a small staff, well-used apparatus, and insufficient funds for major new purchases, but the department's advance in neuroradiology and nuclear medicine, and its special apparatus designed in-house, helped to balance these difficulties.

The Establishment of a Special Studies Section

Procedures in neuroradiology and angiography were begun at the Hospital of the University of Pennsylvania during the 1950s, but they were performed by physicians from the Neurology Department. The Department of Radiology provided equipment and technical assistance and interpreted the films, but it was not until the early 1960s that a radiologist actually became involved in the performance of the procedures.

Mark M. Mishkin became interested in neuroradiology while a departmental resident between 1957 and 1960, and during his residency he was able to spend some time in New York studying these procedures. At Dr. Pendergrass's suggestion he applied for and received a National Institutes of Health fellowship to study abroad and following completion of his residency spent a year studying neuroradiology at the National Hospital, Queen Square, London. Prior to his return home he also had the opportunity to meet the most prominent specialists in neuroradiology in Scandinavia.

[125]

Dr. Mishkin returned to Philadelphia and established a Special Studies Section in the Department of Radiology to perform neuroradiological procedures; the Hospital of the University of Pennsylvania thus became the first hospital in the United States where radiologists performed all of these procedures. Such an operational change had to be handled with special care because, in addition to the matter of professional pride, the neurosurgeons received an estimated $50,000 annually by performing these services. Drs. Pendergrass and Chamberlain took great pains to convince their own and other departments of the importance of this change while Mishkin was in Europe, however, and after only six months of operation had the department's program achieved total acceptance among the hospital's referring physicians.

Mark Mishkin brought the best trained nurse at Queen Square back to Philadelphia with him, and the two of them, with the aid of a technician, ran the entire Special Studies Section. The group designed its own facilities and purchased as much equipment as possible. There were not sufficient funds to purchase all of the apparatus desired, and there was close to a twelve month wait for an image intensifier. Fortunately, they were eventually able to purchase one of the very first portable image intensifiers designed particularly for special procedures in the nation. Dr. Chamberlain was very enthusiastic about this project from its inception, and Dr. Mishkin was given the title of Chief, Special Studies Section, when he returned from abroad.

For the first two years Mishkin concentrated all his efforts in neuroradiology, and his heavy workload precluded much contact with the rest of the department. He continued to be the only staff physician involved with these procedures, but interest among the residents eventually provided him with some additional assistance. The first Fellow specifically assigned to the section, Harry Press, came during the 1964–65 academic year, and in that same year Mishkin began to work in angiography in cooperation with an eminent radiologist, Stanley Baum, who was on the staff at Graduate Hospital.

Demand for these special procedures had increased substantially by 1968, and the decision was made to divide the responsibilities for neuroradiology and angiography. Dr. Mishkin continued as the department's neuroradiologist, and Dr. Arnold Chait, a radiologist at Presbyterian Hospital, came to take over the department's angiography procedures. The Special Studies Section was operated by these two physicians throughout the remainder of Dr. Chamberlain's chairmanship, and Mishkin retained responsibility for neuroradiological procedures at the Hospital of the University of Pennsylvania and Veterans Hospital, as well as at Graduate Hospital, from 1972 to 1975 when he served as Chief of the Department of Radiology at Graduate.[38]

Growth in the Nuclear Medicine Section

David E. Kuhl became a fully-affiliated member of the hospital and University staffs, and Chief of the Nuclear Medicine Section, when he completed his residency program in 1963. At this time the section began to receive grants from the Atomic Energy Commission and the United States Public Health Service to fund special research projects. This established a tradition of substantive outside funding which eventually grew to support the department's machine shop and most of the shop employees. Public Health Service money often included training stipends, which usually provided the section with a postgraduate radiologist or internist to work on its staff. This radiological specialization achieved rapid professional acceptance, and following early accreditation by the American Medical Association its importance quickly reached the point that nuclear medicine facilities, or, in the case of small hospitals, cooperative arrangements with nearby institutions, became a requirement for hospital accreditation by the A.M.A.

David E. Kuhl had pioneered work in nuclear medicine in the 1950s, and in the 1960s he and his staff continued to lead the field. In 1965 they designed and built the first apparatus to perform body section tomography with radionucleotides; tomography itself was a standard procedure, but the utilization of emitted radionucleotides, as opposed to X-rays, was new and proved particularly effective for some diagnostic examinations.

The section's next contribution was in transaxial computed tomography, the very principles which were employed several years later in the development of the EMI Scanner. Kuhl's unit was the first which could record views at various axes; his scanner relied on radionucleotide emissions to create an image, whereas some later apparatus, including the EMI Scanner, relied on transmitted X-ray beams.[39] An even more advanced unit, the Mark IV

Scanner, was installed next to the department's EMI Scanner in 1975, and both units were used in the detailed evaluation of acutely head-injured patients.[40]

The Nuclear Medicine Section concentrated major research efforts on the human brain, and participated in a number of interdisciplinary projects with the hospital's neurologists and neurosurgeons, as well as with independent bodies like the Institute for Neurological Research. The Department of Health, Education and Welfare supported a particularly interesting Head Injury Research Project in an effort to gather substantial amounts of data about patients with this type of injury, especially children, and develop criteria for increasing the accuracy of diagnosis. The project was coordinated by the Office of the Vice President for Medical Affairs, and other institutions were encouraged to send their patients who suffered from head trauma to the department for examination.[41] Other important work in the section involved the body's metabolism, particularly that of the brain. The department's formal tie-in with the Brookhaven Laboratory kept it abreast of the latest work with radioactive compounds and enabled it to utilize new compounds shortly after they became available. Work with new computers and algorithms helped to improve scanning techniques and image construction.

This extensive research program, plus ongoing diagnostic work, was carried out in increasingly cramped facilities, and by the end of Dr. Chamberlain's chairmanship much additional space was needed by the section.[42] Happily, David E. Kuhl's outstanding contributions to nuclear medicine were appropriately recognized when he was honored in the spring of 1976 with the Nuclear Pioneer Citation from the Society of Nuclear Medicine.

Operation of the Departments of Radiology at the Veterans Administration Hospital and Graduate Hospital

The proximity of the University of Pennsylvania School of Medicine to a number of large, metropolitan hospitals greatly increased the variety of clinical rotations available to its students. Similarly, area hospitals which needed additional staffing and expertise often called upon the School of Medicine for assistance. Such was the case when the Veterans Administration Hospital became an affiliated teaching hospital in the early 1960s.

Unlike most of the specialty departments at the V.A. at this time, however, their Department of Radiology was self-sustaining and fully operative, so it was entirely inappropriate for the staff at the Hospital of the University of Pennsylvania and the School of Medicine to interfere in the operation. Its position deteriorated considerably throughout the decade, however, and in May, 1969, against Dr. Chamberlain's wishes, he became responsible for the entire operation.[43]

The facilities at the V.A. were old and outdated, so the first priority was an extensive remodeling and re-equipping of the hospital's diagnostic facilities. The hospital had its own radiotherapy apparatus, and with the installation of a new cobalt therapy unit shortly after the reorganization its therapy case load began to show a healthy increase.[44] An entirely new neuroradiology suite was also installed.[45] In addition to its own staff, physicians from the Hospital of the University of Pennsylvania rotated through the V.A. Its status as a teaching institution permitted the rotation of residents through the department and gave the undergraduate medical students the opportunity to observe and study.[46]

Graduate Hospital, on the other hand, was wholly owned by the University of Pennsylvania (it was originally the teaching hospital for the Graduate School of Medicine), and many of its staff radiologists were members of the faculty of the School of Medicine, as were the staff radiologists at the Hospital of the University of Pennsylvania. The existence of these two separate Departments of Radiology within the School of Medicine was somewhat further complicated by faculty representation from two other affiliated teaching hospitals, Presbyterian-University of Pennsylvania Medical Center and Pennsylvania Hospital.

In October, 1972, during a period of University and community concern about the future of Graduate Hospital, Dr. Chamberlain was named Director of its Department of Radiology. In many respects this produced benefits for the School of Medicine: there was now a single department, and the opportunities to share staff expertise, materials, and services, and thereby improve teaching, research, and patient care, were markedly enhanced. There were also enormous administrative difficulties, particularly in view of Dr. Chamberlain's complex financial arrangements with the hospital and University.[47]

Dr. Chamberlain appointed Mark M. Mishkin as Chief of the department at Graduate, but Mishkin also retained his responsibility for the neuroradiology program at HUP and the V.A.[48] The department at Graduate operated as a subdivision of the department at HUP; patients were charged on the same fee schedules, and residents served regular rotations there. This rotation proved particularly valuable because it exposed the residents to a nonacademic setting, and the staff at Graduate was stimulated by its contact with these young physicians.[49]

As at the V.A., one of the first priorities for the operation at Graduate was a detailed plan for the total remodeling of its facilities. Included were examination and special procedure rooms, as well as facilities for nuclear medicine. Therapeutic consultations were done at Graduate, but patients were referred to HUP for their actual treatment.[50]

The formal combination of radiologic operations at these three hospitals was particularly valuable for the Nuclear Medicine Section, because it was able to expand its range of services in each institution through the sharing of staff. A joint radiopharmaceutical laboratory was established to distribute short-lived radionucleotides to each hospital each morning; such an operation increased efficiency while lowering the cost. As the section added more procedures, additional equipment was installed at each institution.[51]

After many years of discussion, the University Trustees and Graduate Hospital established an independent Board of Managers at Graduate, and the radiology services were separated in July, 1975. Dr. Arnold Chait, a radiologist at HUP, was eventually chosen to head the Department of Radiology at Graduate Hospital.

Throughout this period the relationship between the Departments of Radiology at the Hospital of the University of Pennsylvania and the Veterans Administration Hospital remained the same, and the final phase of the overall expansion at the V.A. was completed by the construction of a research building. New fluoroscopic rooms came about as a result of the research building construction, and in 1975 an angiography unit and a unit for body section radiology were installed. Following the termination of the University's teaching arrangement with the University of Saigon, Dr. James T. Lambeth, the radiologist who had run the program in Vietnam, came to Philadelphia to head up the department at the Veterans Administration Hospital.[52]

Changes in the Residency Program

The residency program was four years long in 1961. Three years were devoted to diagnostic radiology, including a three month concentration on neuroradiology and angiography. Nine months were devoted to therapeutic radiology, and three months to nuclear medicine. During these rotations, and particularly while they were studying general diagnostic radiology, residents were given considerable responsibility for decision making and general department operation. Instruction was often informal; this was possible because there was a small staff and a small group of residents studying in the department each year. Residents were responsible for "walking the floor": speaking to patients, deciding which views to take, following-up on patients as they moved through the department, and checking films for technical accuracy in the control room.[53]

As the number of residents and the workload increased, however, it became impossible for each resident to review all the cases each day. Residents still dictated reports on ward patients, which were checked by senior physicians the following day, but it was necessary to eliminate much of the time formerly spent by residents in joint case review with senior staff members. Many junior residents learned a great deal of fluoroscopy by observing the more senior members of their ranks. By 1970, specialization within radiology had increased so greatly that the department created separate diagnostic and therapeutic residencies and reduced the period of study to three years.[54]

With the increased specialization in the residency training program, the physicians were less willing to learn by observing senior staff members or senior residents, and before they were given responsibility for handling various procedures they wanted formal instruction, lectures, and conferences. This increased emphasis on formal instruction, particularly in personalized instruction for various procedures, was accompanied by greater exposure to pathology. Residents were given less responsibility for decision making. They read films with senior physicians, but did not have the opportunity to read them beforehand and benefit later from the comments and critique of senior staff members. Only at the Veterans Administration Hospital did the residents continue to function fairly independently.[55]

Residents in the diagnostic program took formal courses in the Graduate School of Medicine during their first and third years, and also participated in daily teaching and clinical conferences and weekly specialty conferences which highlighted a specific field, such as neuroradiology or abdominal angiography. They attended a special four week course in nuclear medicine[56] and were also given instruction in radiophysics and radiobiology. Residents in the therapy program participated in joint hospital conferences with physicians from the Departments of Medicine, Surgery, Gynecology, and Otorhinolaryngology. They were also given formal instruction in areas of special interest in advanced radiotherapy, but received most of their fundamental instruction by working with senior physicians and patients.[57]

For many years the Department of Radiology at HUP had operated its own residency program, while the departments at Presbyterian and Graduate operated a joint program. The realignment in the School of Medicine necessitated a change in this organization, however, and the American Medical Association approved a combined program, for HUP, Graduate, and the V.A. as of July 1, 1973, and the establishment of an independent residency at Presbyterian-University of Pennsylvania Medical Center.[58]

The increasing specialization within the discipline of radiology was clearly seen in the creation of two separate residency programs at the Hospital of the University of Pennsylvania and its affiliated institutions. It is also apparent in the insistence by residents that they receive formal instruction in the various aspects of their specializations.

Changes in the School of Medicine Curriculum

Radiology course offerings gradually increased in number in the School of Medicine, another clear indication of specialization within the discipline. Richard Chamberlain insisted that a basic course in radiology be required as part of the medical school curriculum, and despite some arguments from other members of the faculty, a requirement was instituted. The course was offered near the end of the first year of course work, after the students had had a minimum of exposure to radiology in their anatomy, pathology, medicine, and surgery courses, and was designed to expose students to the fundamental concepts of diagnostic and therapeutic radiology and nuclear medicine through lectures, demonstrations, and small group conferences.[59]

The expansion of course offerings was spearheaded by Wallace T. Miller, a departmental Fellow during the late 1950s, who returned to the hospital following his military service as one of the small staff of diagnosticians. His informal case reviews were an ever popular offering, and his enthusiasm for and commitment to undergraduate medical education were reflected by his receipt of the Lindback Award for Distinguished Teaching in 1968, the Student Government Teaching Award in 1972, and the dedication of the 1971 medical school yearbook to Miller and three other physicians.

Adele K. Friedman, another diagnostic radiologist, accepted specific responsibility for the expanded general radiology elective,[60] and it grew to become so popular that seventy-five percent of the medical students took it sometime during their four years in school.[61] The course was taught as a preceptorship with daily interpretive film conferences as well as lectures, demonstrations, and joint conferences with other specialties. Fluoroscopy, special studies, and nuclear medicine were included in the curriculum, with special attention to the use of radionucleotides.[62]

The expanded list of advanced course offerings included pediatric radiology, clinical diagnosis, gastrointestinal radiology, and two courses in radiological physics.[63] A four week clinical nuclear medicine course, taught each January, was particularly popular. Exposure to radiotherapy for the undergraduate medical student was confined primarily to information in the introductory courses and a single course in therapeutic radiology.[64]

Advances in diagnostic and therapeutic radiology increased its value to other specialists considerably during these years. The importance of an understanding of the capabilities of radiologic techniques was stressed to students in the School of Medicine, and the expanded offerings enabled the interested student to receive more in-depth exposure to one or more facets of the radiological program.

Richard H. Chamberlain's Outside Activities

In addition to his responsibilities as Chairman of the Department of Radiology, Richard Chamberlain was appointed to a number of international committees, was active in radiological and medical organizations, and developed a number of projects which involved the department outside the hospital. Among the most extensive of these were teaching assistance to the University of Saigon and creation of the Radiation Management Corporation.

Chamberlain was a recognized expert on radiation units and measurements, and served on a number of international commissions charged with the analysis of exposure to radiation and its effect. He served on the World Health Organization's Expert Advisory Panel on Radiation for ten years, lectured for that organization on radiation health in the eastern Mediterranean, western Pacific, and southeast Asia, and served as a member of several other of its committees. During his trips to southeast Asia, he became acutely conscious of the lack of a strong radiological teaching program in that part of the world. His interest in this problem prompted him to enter into a contract with the American Medical Association and the United States Agency for International Development to maintain an interdepartmental relationship with the Department of Radiology at the University of Saigon.

After a preliminary visit in 1969, Dr. Chamberlain was able to outline a number of problems at three teaching hospitals in Saigon: deficiencies in the number of professional and technical personnel, inappropriate selection and poor maintenance of equipment, and lack of understanding of—or attention to—quality control in radiograph production.[65] He visited the departments in Saigon once or twice a year to observe their progress, but chose Dr. James T. Lambeth, a radiologist from the University of California, to supervise the on-site operation.[66] Lambeth oversaw the residency in radiology, presented lectures on diagnostic radiology to medical students, and planned a training program for technicians. The latter was designed to familiarize them with up-to-date apparatus prior to their being sent to district health units, but, as with other planned programs, political instability often intervened.[67] Each of the Chiefs of Radiology at the teaching hospitals came to Philadelphia to complete an advanced course of study at the Hospital of the University of Pennsylvania, as did other Vietnamese physicians: thirty-one completed one year of specialized training and six completed two years of specialized training.[68]

Once Vietnamese personnel were properly trained, however, they still faced difficulties with the apparatus available for their use. Richard Chamberlain was particularly conscious of the need for a manageable, streamlined diagnostic system which could operate under primitive conditions in rural areas, and which could be used effectively by technical personnel without extensive training. To meet these needs he developed the Technamatic Radiology System, a battery-operated unit which offered a limited number of exposure settings and body positions and used special film, to compensate for the area's high humidity, which was processed inside the unit.[69] The system was marketed by the General Electric Company and created worldwide interest because its cost was reasonable, it assured high quality films, and it reduced the technician's responsibility for decision making.[70]

Two Technamatic units were installed in Saigon teaching hospitals, in addition to new conventional apparatus in eight examination rooms. The Technamatic system was used by the hospital staffs, but political unrest prevented thorough training programs for medical students and technologists.[71] The cooperative program with the University of Saigon came to an abrupt halt in 1975; by that time nine Technamatic units had been installed in Vietnam.[72] Despite the system's technical efficiency, it was destined to fail in the Third World because there was no prestige associated with the ownership of such a simplistic piece of apparatus.[73]

Richard Chamberlain also served as a consultant to a number of national organizations, including the National Advisory Council on Radiation and the National Council on Radiation Protection, and was an active participant in the work of University committees and local and state medical societies and organizations. As a member of the State of Pennsylvania Advisory Committee on Atomic Energy, he interacted with responsible officials from business, industry, and state government, and found that there was extreme concern about the industrial uses of radiation and the potential for a disaster.

With the assistance of a local Philadelphia businessman, Dr. Chamberlain organized the Radiation Management Corporation in 1969. The effort was funded by the sale of stock shares among industrial users in the mid-Atlantic region, and its purpose was to pursue research on the evaluation, diagnosis, and treatment of all types of radiation exposure. Dr. Roger E. Linnemann, a respected specialist in radiological protection, left the U.S. Army to become President of the corporation. It was responsible for the laboratory and nonclinical aspects of the investigation, while the department was responsible for the clinical aspects of the program.

The department equipped a residential treatment center on the sixth floor of the Maloney Building, incuding a radiosurgery decontamination room and a reverse isolation room. Hospital personnel were trained to handle radiation emergencies, and the corporation and department jointly maintained surface and air transportation which could respond immediately in the case of an emergency. The corporation's independent status enabled it to fund special projects at the hospital, and in the early 1970s it funded the Department of Hematology so that it could use the special clinical facility for a bone marrow transplant program, and donated a laminar air reverse isolation room for the clinical facility as well as a centrifuge for the Blood Bank. Dr. Linnemann held a faculty appointment, and the corporation's staff also participated in programs for medical students and residents.[74]

Richard H. Chamberlain's enthusiastic commitment to projects outside the hospital, in addition to his work at the hospital and School of Medicine, earned him respect among radiologists worldwide. He was honored with the receipt of the Gold Medal of the American College of Radiology in 1969, the Gold Medal of the Radiological Society of North America in 1971, and the Medal of the University of Lund, Sweden in 1975.

NOTES

1. Edward M. DeYoung, Personal Interview, 7 June 1978.
2. Hospital of the University of Pennsylvania, *Annual Report of the Board of Managers* (31 May 1953), p. 36.
3. DeYoung, Personal Interview, 7 June 1978.
4. *Ibid.*
5. Mark M. Mishkin, Personal Interview, Spring 1976; Wallace T. Miller, Personal Interview, Spring 1976; Larissa T. Bilaniuk, Personal Interview, Spring 1976.
6. Adele K. Friedman, Personal Interview, Spring 1976.
7. Mishkin, Personal Interview, Spring 1976.

8. Friedman, Personal Interview, Spring 1976.

9. DeYoung, Personal Interview, 7 June 1978; Mishkin, Personal Interview, Spring 1976.

10. Miller, Personal Interview, Spring 1976.

11. DeYoung, Personal Interview, 7 June 1978.

12. Miller, Personal Interview, Spring 1976.

13. Friedman, Personal Interview, Spring 1976.

14. Bilaniuk, Personal Interview, Spring 1976.

15. Hospital of the University of Pennsylvania, *Annual Report* (30 June 1965), inside front cover.

16. Hospital of the University of Pennsylvania, *Annual Report* (30 June 1968), p. 27.

17. Hospital of the University of Pennsylvania, *Annual Report* (30 June 1971), p. 10; Friedman, Personal Interview, Spring 1976; Mishkin, Personal Interview, Spring 1976.

18. *University of Pennsylvania Medical Center Biennial Report, 1971–73* (Philadelphia: 1973), p. 193.

19. Bilaniuk, Personal Interview, Spring 1976.

20. Eugene P. Pendergrass, Personal Interview, 17 June 1976; Hospital of the University of Pennsylvania, *Annual Report,* 1965, p. 25; "The Wilson Professorship," *Medical Affairs* II, No. 3 (1961): 28–29.

21. *University of Pennsylvania Medical Center Annual Report, 1970–71* (Philadelphia: 1971), p. 142.

22. *Biennial Report,* p. 194.   23. *Ibid.,* p. 195.

24. *Ibid.*   25. *Annual Report,* 1970–71, pp. 143–44.

26. *Biennial Report,* p. 195.

27. Friedman, Personal Interview, Spring 1976; Bilaniuk, Personal Interview, Spring 1976.

28. *Annual Report,* p. 139.

29. *Biennial Report,* p. 193.

30. DeYoung, Personal Interview, 7 June 1978.

31. Miller, Personal Interview, Spring 1976.

32. DeYoung, Personal Interview, 7 June 1978; Mishkin, Personal Interview, Spring 1976.

33. DeYoung, Personal Interview, 7 June 1978.

34. Mishkin, Personal Interview, Spring 1976.

35. *Ibid.*

36. Richard H. Chamberlain to Alfred A. Gellhorn, 22 May 1972, Department of Radiology Records and Registers, Miscellaneous Papers, Hospital of the University of Pennsylvania, Philadelphia.

37. *Annual Report,* 1970–71, p. 144.

38. Mishkin, Personal Interview, Spring 1976.

39. David E. Kuhl, Personal Interview, 10 March 1976.

40. *University of Pennsylvania Medical Center Triennial Report 1973–76* (Philadelphia: 1976), p. 260.

41. Kuhl, Personal Interview, 10 March 1976; *Triennial Report,* p. 257.

42. Kuhl, Personal Interview, 10 March 1976.

43. DeYoung, Personal Interview, 7 June 1978.

44. *Annual Report,* p. 139.

45. *Biennial Report,* p. 193.

46. DeYoung, Personal Interview, 7 June 1978.

47. *Biennial Report,* p. 190.

48. *Ibid.*

49. Mishkin, Personal Interview, Spring 1976.

50. *Biennial Report,* p. 193.

51. *Ibid.,* p. 194.

52. *Triennial Report,* pp. 255–56.

53. Bilaniuk, Personal Interview, Spring 1976.

54. *Ibid.*   55. *Ibid.*

56. *Annual Report,* p. 141.   57. *Biennial Report,* p. 192.

58. *Ibid.*

59. *Annual Report,* p. 140; Miller, Personal Interview, Spring 1976.

60. Miller, Personal Interview, Spring 1976.

61. *Biennial Report,* p. 192.

62. *Ibid.; University of Pennsylvania Bulletin: School of Medicine* **77**, No. 10 (1977–78) (Philadelphia: 1976): 82.

63. *Bulletin:* 82.   64. *Biennial Report,* p. 192.

65. *Annual Report,* p. 141.

66. DeYoung, Personal Interview, 7 June 1978.

67. *Biennial Report,* p. 193.

68. *Ibid,* p. 259.

69. DeYoung, Personal Interview, 7 June 1978.

70. *Annual Report,* p. 142.

71. *Biennial Report,* p. 192.

72. *Triennial Report,* p. 259.

73. DeYoung, Personal Interview, 7 June 1978.

74. *Ibid.; Annual Report,* p. 142; *Biennial Report,* p. 196.

A Look Toward the Future

Stanley Baum

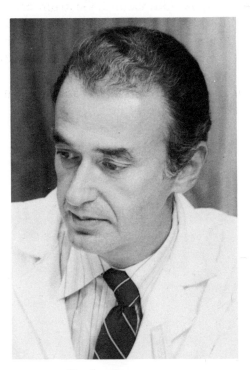

Stanley Baum, 1975

In July of 1975, Dr. Stanley Baum, a pioneer in vascular radiology, was appointed Professor and Chairman of the Department of Radiology. Because of ill health, Dr. Richard H. Chamberlain retired from the administrative duties of the Department of Radiology, but he remained Professor until his untimely death in December of the same year.

It was Dr. Baum's view that the specialty of radiation therapy had progressed to the point where it should stand as a separate department within the School of Medicine and hospital, and at his request the University Provost, Dean of the School of Medicine, and University Long-Range Planning Committee agreed to establish an independent department. A search committee was organized to find someone to head this department, and in July, 1977 Dr. Robert L. Goodman came to Pennsylvania to head the new Department of Radiation Therapy.

Under Dr. Baum's direction the Department of Radiology was divided into diagnostic radiology and nuclear medicine. Diagnostic radiology in turn was sectionalized into Angiography, Computerized Tomography/Ultrasound, Gastrointestinal, Genitourinary, Neuroradiology, Orthopedic, Out Patient, Pulmonary, and Radiological Physics. Each section was staffed with radiologists whose major academic interests were in these specific areas. Radiology at Pennsylvania had made giant advances since Charles Lester Leonard's one room operation, and it would continue to lead its field in the years to come.

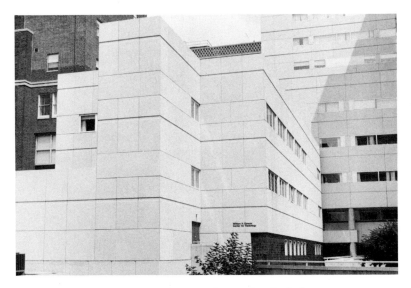

William H. Donner Center for Radiology

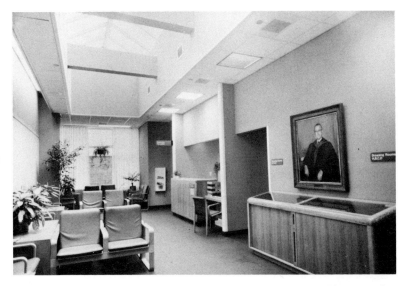

*Reception area of the Eugene P. Pendergrass Outpatient Clinic at the
Radiology Department*

Appendix

EXPLANATORY NOTE: The compilation of a comprehensive personnel listing for the Department of Radiology is not possible because records are not available for the period when the operation was independent from the hospital. Moreover, semantic differences with respect to titles appear regularly throughout the available records.

The *Annual Reports of the Board of Managers,* and subsequent hospital *Annual Reports,* were chosen as the source for this appendix because they cover the entire period from 1899 to 1973. There are, however, omissions and difficulties even with these records. Their personnel lists include only those individuals working at University Hospital. The names of persons working at other institutions, with appointments in the School of Medicine, do not appear. Nurses, technicians, and other auxiliary staff members are not included after 1941. The years cited refer to the date of the report; the hospital's fiscal year ended variously in May, June, August, and December during this period. Such dating is particularly frustrating when an appointment made in July does not appear until the report of the following spring. Perhaps the greatest weakness, however, is the closing date of 1973: no comparable sources exist for the period 1973 to date to permit the inclusion of additional names, nor the updating of titles.

Care should be taken not to use this appendix as an absolute reference to date departmental activities. Even with its problems, however, it will be useful for quick reference.

Personnel in the Department of Radiology, Hospital of the University of Pennsylvania, 1899–1973, as listed in the *Annual Report of the Board of Managers* (1899–1963) and *Annual Report* (1964–1973).

Abercrombie, Eugene M.D.— 1924–25
   Roentgenologic Interne Acinapura, Yolanda—Therapy

Technician 1936–37;
Diagnostic Technician
1938–39

Ackerman, Joseph L. M.D.—
Resident 1955

Alavi, Abass M.D.—Resident
1972–73

Alexander, Fay Knight M.D.—
Fellow in Radiology (Resident)
1931–32; Fellow in Radiology
1933–35

Allen, Kenneth A. M.D.—
Roentgenologic Interne 1925

Allen, M. Lowry M.D.—Fellow
in Radiology 1932–33

Allen, William R. M.D.—
Resident 1948

Andrews, J. Robert M.D.—
Resident in Radiology 1934–35

Arger, Peter H. M.D.—Associate
in Radiology 1970–73

Asmino, M. M.D.—Resident
1956; House Staff 1957–58

Atkins, Harold L. M.D.—
Resident 1954; Heublein
Fellow 1955; American Cancer
Society (National
Organization) Fellow 1956

Ayella, Robert J. M.D.—Resident
1950–51

Barcena-Jannet, Roberto M.D.—
Resident 1970–73

Barden, Robert P. M.D.—
Resident in Radiology 1936;
Fellow in Radiology and
Assistant Instructor 1937–38;
Associate in Radiology
1942–49; Visiting Radiologist
1962–73

Barden, Stuart P. M.D.—
Resident in Radiology
1942–44

Barnes, Maurine Reed M.D.—
Associate in Radiology
1964–69

Bartlett, Clara R.N.—Nurse and
Technician 1925–28; Nurse
Technician 1929

Bassols, Francisco M.D.—
Resident 1945

Bavendam, Frederick A. M.D.—
Resident 1946

Baxter, Thomas F. M.D.—
Roentgenologic Interne 1924

Bearor, Robert A. M.D.—House
Staff 1961–62; Trainee,
National Cancer Institute
1961–62; American Cancer
Society (National
Organization) Fellow 1962

Becker, Joseph M. M.D.—
Resident 1972–73

Benson, John M. M.D.—
Resident 1972–73

Berger, Raymond A. M.D.—
Fellow in Radiology
1935–36

Berry, Harrison M. D.D.S.—
Associate, Dental
Roentgenology 1964–73

Bilaniuk, Larissa T. M.D.—
Resident 1967–71; Associate in
Radiology 1972–73

Billiet, Ignace M.D.—
Departmental Resident 1964

Bledsoe, Theodore R. M.D.—
House Staff 1962; American
Cancer Society (Philadelphia
Division) Fellow 1962;
Departmental Resident
1964–65

Bloch, Peter Ph.D.—Radiological
Physicist 1969–73

Blount, Henry C. M.D.—
Resident 1950; DuPont Fellow
1951–52; Resident 1953

Bluth, Edward I. M.D.—Resident
1972–73

Booth, Robert E. M.D.—
Resident 1945–46

Borns, Patricia M.D.—DuPont
Fellow 1953; American Cancer
Society (Philadelphia Division)
Fellow 1954; DuPont Fellow
1955

Boudreau, Robert P. M.D.—
Resident 1951; American
Cancer Society (Philadelphia
Division) Fellow 1952; Damon
Runyon Fellow (American
Cancer Society) 1953; Trainee,
National Cancer Institute 1954

Boyer, John L. M.D.—Resident
1945–46

Brackin, John T. Jr. M.D.—
Resident and Assistant
Instructor in Radiology 1939;
Fellow and Assistant Instructor
1940–41

Brady, Luther W. Jr. M.D.—
Trainee, National Cancer
Institute 1956–57; Associate in
Radiology 1957–59

Brennan, James T. M.D.—
Associate in Radiology
1967–73

Brindle, Harry R. M.D.—Fellow
in Radiology 1937

Briney, Allan K. M.D.—Resident
1949; Trainee, National Cancer
Institute 1950–52

Brooks, Frank P. M.D.—Resident
1945–46

Brown, George H. M.D.—
Resident and Assistant
Instructor in Radiology 1940;
Fellow and Assistant Instructor
1941; Fellow 1942; Resident
1943

Burt, Robert W. M.D.—Resident
1970–73

Bustamente, José P. M.D.—
Resident 1969–71

Butler, Horace G. M.D.—
Resident 1948–49; DuPont

Fellow 1950; Pennsylvania
Manufacturers Association
Fellow 1950; Visiting
Radiologist 1960–64

Byrne, Robert N. M.D.—
Resident 1949

Campbell, Robert E. M.D.—
House Staff 1959–61;
Pennsylvania Manufacturers
Association Fellow 1960;
American Cancer Society
(National Organization) Fellow
1961–62; Associate in
Radiology 1962

Campoy, Francisco M.D.—
Resident 1950; American
Cancer Society (Philadelphia
Division) Fellow 1951;
Heublein Fellow 1952;
Resident 1953

Card, Richard Y. M.D.—
Resident 1956

Carrasco, Cesar M.D.—House
Staff 1960–61

Casselman, Edward S. M.D.—
Resident 1972–73

Chait, Arnold M.D.—Associate
in Radiology 1970–73

Chamberlain, George W. M.D.—
Fellow in Radiology 1935;
Associate in Radiology 1936;
Associate in Radiology and
Instructor in Radiology
1937–41

Chamberlain, Richard H. M.D.—
Resident and Assistant
Instructor 1941; Fellow 1942;
Resident, 1943; Associate in
Radiology 1946–52;
Therapeutic Division:
Professor of Radiology
1953–61; Assistant Director of
the Donner Center 1959–61;
Chairman and Director of the
Donner Center 1962–73

Chandler, Dick E. M.D.—House
Staff 1957

Chavez, Ignacio M.D.—Resident
1956; House Staff 1957;
Pennsylvania Manufacturers
Association Fellow 1958

Chen, James T. M.D.—House
Staff 1957 and 1961–62;
Department of Radiology
Fund Fellow 1961–62

Chiappori, Miguel M.D.—House
Staff 1958–61; DuPont Fellow
1960; Heublein Fellow 1961

Chon, Hikon M.D.—Resident
1969–71; Associate in
Radiology 1972–73

Citro, Lawrence A. M.D.—
Resident 1971–73

Cocke, John A. M.D.—Resident
1946–47; Trainee, National
Cancer Institute 1948

Cohoon, Carl W. M.D.—
Roentgenologic Resident
Physician 1928; Resident
Physician 1929

Conway, James J. M.D.—
Departmental Resident
1965–69

Corkle, Robert F. M.D.—
Resident 1950–51

Crow, Harte C. M.D.—
Departmental Resident
1964–66 and 1968; Associate
in Radiology 1969–73

Cynn, Won S. M.D.—Associate
in Radiology 1972–73

Dann, Robert H. Jr. M.D.—
Departmental Resident 1966
and 1969–70; Associate in
Radiology 1971–73

Daryavaz, Ismet M.D.—Resident
1967–69

Daughtridge, T. Griffin M.D.—
Associate in Radiology

1964–66; Visiting Radiologist
1972–73

Davis, Dorothy W. R.N.—Nurse
and Technician 1926–31;
Technician 1932–35;
Diagnostic Technician
1936–41

Davis, Lawrence W. M.D.—
Departmental Resident
1964–66; Associate in
Radiology 1968–73

Deak, Olga R.N.—Nurse
Technician 1930–31

de LaFlor, Jorge M.D.—Resident
1948–49

de Moor, Jacques M.D.—
Heublein Fellow 1953–54;
DuPont Fellow 1954; Heublein
Fellow 1955

Dennis, John M. M.D.—
Heublein Fellow 1951–52

DePoto, Donald W. M.D.—
Resident 1967–71

Devenney, John E. M.D.—
Resident 1972–73

Devitt, William M.D.—Assistant
in X-Ray Department
1909–10

DeYoung, Edward M. M.D.—
Resident 1947; Associate in
Radiology 1962–73

Doyle, A. S. M.D.—Assistant
Roentgenologist 1916–22

Dziamski, Marian M.D.—House
Staff 1962

Eaton, Walter L. Jr. M.D.—
House Staff 1961–62; Trainee,
National Cancer Institute
1962; Pennsylvania
Manufacturers Association
Fellow 1962; Departmental
Resident 1964; Associate in
Radiology 1967–73

Eby, Charles E. M.D.—Resident

1952; Trainee, National Cancer Institute 1953

Echeverri, Alvaro F. M.D.—House Staff 1960

Edeiken, Jack M.D.—Resident 1949; Trainee, National Cancer Institute 1950–51; Resident 1952; Associate in Radiology 1954–58

Ennis, LeRoy M. D.D.S.—Consultant Dental Radiologist 1943–49

Ernst, Richard E. M.D.—Resident 1955; Heublein Fellow 1956; Trainee, National Cancer Institute 1957; Pennsylvania Manufacturers Association Fellow 1957

Essinger, Axel R. M.D.—House Staff 1962; Heublein Fellow 1962

Eyler, Paul W. M.D.—Resident 1947; Trainee, National Cancer Institute 1948; Resident 1949; Associate in Radiology 1950–51

Eymontt, Michael J. M.D.—Resident 1971; Associate in Radiology 1972–73

Factor, Donald E. M.D.—Resident 1969–73

Farley, Hal D. M.D.—Departmental Resident 1964–65

Farrell, Corinne M.D.—House Staff 1961–62; Trainee, National Cancer Institute 1962; Departmental Resident 1964

Fencel, Richard M. M.D.—House Staff 1962; Trainee, National Cancer Institute 1962; Resident 1965–66; Associate in Radiology 1967

Fenton, Craig A. M.D.—Resident 1972–73

Finkelstein, Arthur K. M.D.—Visiting Radiologist 1966–71; Associate in Radiology 1972–73

Finkelstein, Leah Shore M.D.—Associate in Radiology 1972–73

Fitz, Charles R. M.D.—Resident 1967–71

Foley, Eugene F. M.D.—House Staff 1960–62; Trainee, National Cancer Institute 1961–62, Associate in Radiology 1964–65

Forbes, Thomas W. M.D.—Resident 1972–73

Forsted, David H. M.D.—Resident 1972–73

Fortney, Jeanne—Technician 1935

Fox, Henry J. M.D.—Resident 1954–55; Trainee, National Cancer Institute 1956

Freed, John H. M.D.—Resident 1946–48; Associate in Radiology 1949–50

Friedlander, Milton A. M.D.—House Staff 1961–62; Trainee, National Cancer Institute 1962; DuPont Fellow 1962; Departmental Resident 1964

Friedman, Adele Kynette M.D.—Associate in Radiology 1957–73 (See KYNETTE)

Garrahan, C. Justus, M.S.—Technician 1933–35; Physicist 1936–37

George, David Ph.D.—Radiological Physicist 1969–73

Gibbons, John F. M.D.—Resident 1950; Damon

Runyon Fellow (American
Cancer Society) 1951–52;
Resident 1953

Godfrey, Ellwood W. M.D.—
Resident and Assistant
Instructor in Radiology 1939;
Fellow and Assistant Instructor
1940–41; Fellow 1942;
Resident 1943

Goldmark, Peter C. Ph.D.—
Visiting Professor of Medical
Electronics 1951–62

Gordon, Michael E. M.D.—
Resident 1971–73

Gorson, Robert O. M.S.—
Physicist 1953–59

Graham, Gladwyn D.D.S.—
Consultant in Dental
Radiology 1955–59

Graves, A. Judson M.D.—
Resident in Radiology 1938;
Fellow and Assistant Instructor
in Radiology 1939–40

Grawl, Marian Rust—Technician
1934–35; Therapy Technician
1936–37

Greaves, Harrison H. M.D.—
Assistant in X-Ray Laboratory
1911; Assistant
Roentgenologist 1912–15

Greening, Roy R. M.D.—
Resident 1949; Damon
Runyon Fellow (American
Cancer Society) 1950;
Associate in Radiology
1951–58; School of Nursing
Faculty 1958

Grippe, William J. M.D.—
Resident 1952; Trainee,
National Cancer Institute
1953–54

Gureghian, Patricia A. M.D.—
Associate in Radiology
1972–73

Hale, John Ph.D.—Radiologic

Physicist 1950–73

Hall, Wendell C. M.D.—Fellow
in Radiology (Resident) 1933;
Fellow in Radiology 1934–35

Hansell, John R. M.D.—
Associate in Radiology
1972–73

Hansen, Alton S. M.D.—
Resident 1946–47

Harris, John Jr. M.D.—Visiting
Radiologist 1959–61

Harris, John H. M.D.—Fellow in
Radiology 1934–35

Harris, John H. M.D.—Resident
1955; Trainee, National Cancer
Institute 1956–57

Harrison, Frank S. M.D.—
Resident 1966

Hay, Percy D., Jr. M.D.—
Roentgenologic Resident
Physician 1928

Hayes, David F. M.D.—Resident
1972–73

Hayes, Thomas P. M.D.—
Resident 1969–71

Hepler, Thomas R. M.D.—
Resident 1952; American
Cancer Society (Philadelphia
Division) Fellow 1953;
Pennsylvania Manufacturers
Association Fellow 1954

Herasme, Victor M. M.D.—
Resident 1972–73

Heublein, Gilbert W. M.D.—
Fellow in Radiology 1937;
Fellow in Radiology and
Assistant Instructor 1938–39

Hillman, David C. M.D.—House
Staff 1962; Trainee, National
Cancer Institute 1962;
Departmental Resident
1965–67

Hirschfeld, Robert L. M.D.—
Associate in Radiology
1965–66

Hodes, Philip J. M.D.—Fellow in Radiology 1934–35; Associate in Radiology 1936; Associate in Radiology and Instructor in Radiology 1937–41; Associate in Radiology 1942–52; Diagnostic Division: Professor of Radiology 1953–58

Hoffert, Paul W. M.D.—Resident 1949

Hope, John W. M.D.—Resident 1948–49; Trainee, National Cancer Institute 1950; Associate in Radiology 1951

Houser, L. Murray M.D.—House Staff 1957; Trainee, National Cancer Institute 1958–60; Associate in Radiology 1961

Huang, Shih-Chang M.D.—Resident 1950–52

Isard, Harold J. M.D.—Visiting Staff 1950–51

Jacobs, Robert M.D.—House Staff 1958–61; American Cancer Society (Philadelphia Division) Fellow 1959–60; Trainee, National Cancer Institute 1961

Jamison, John H. M.D.—Resident in Radiology 1937; Fellow in Radiology and Assistant Instructor 1938–39

Jamison, W. R. M.D.—Technician, Roentgenology 1924–29 (alternate spelling: JAMIESON)

Jarvis, J. Luther M.D.—Resident 1951–52

Jezic, Dragen V. M.D.—Departmental Resident 1965–68

Johnson, Vincent C. M.D.—Fellow in Roentgenology (Resident) 1930; Fellow in Radiology 1931

Jung, Walter K. M.D.—Resident 1970–73

Kaplan, Carl M.D.—House Staff 1959–60; Trainee, National Cancer Institute 1960

Katterjohn, James C. M.D.—Resident 1946–47; Trainee, National Cancer Institute 1948

Keefer, George Pfahler M.D.—Resident and Assistant Instructor 1941; Fellow 1942; Resident 1943

Kern, John D. M.D.—Departmental Resident 1965–68

Kim, San Soo M.D.—Resident 1968–71

King, Lois I. M.D.—DuPont Fellow 1952; Trainee, National Cancer Institute 1953

Kirsh, David M.D.—Resident 1943–46

Klempfner, George M.D.—Resident 1969–70

Konn, Fayetta I. R.N.—Technician 1933–35; Diagnostic Technician 1936–38

Kornblum, Karl M.D.—Assistant Chief of Clinic and Instructor in Surgery 1928–30; Instructor in Radiology 1931–34; Associate in Radiology 1943–44

Kuhl, David E. M.D.—House Staff 1959–61; American Cancer Society Fellow 1960–61; Associate in Radiology 1962–73; School of Nursing Faculty 1962

Kusner, David B.S.—Physicist 1958–61

Ky, Le Dinh M.D.—Resident 1972–73

Kynette, L. Adele M.D.—
Resident 1952; Trainee,
National Cancer Institute
1953–55; Associate in
Radiology 1955–56 (see
FRIEDMAN)

Lafferty, John O. M.D.—
Resident 1944 and 1947;
Trainee, National Cancer
Institute 1948, Resident 1949

Lame, Edwin L. M.D.—Resident
1943–44; Associate in
Radiology 1945–47; Visiting
Radiologist 1966

Laszlo, Arthur M. M.D.—
Resident 1970–73

Lebo, Christine M. R.N.—Nurse
and Technician 1926–31;
Technician 1932–35; Therapy
Technician 1936–41

Lenna, Babette H. M.D.—
Resident 1967–71

Leonard, Charles L. M.D.—
Skiagrapher 1899–1901

Limeaoco, Vicente R. M.D.—
Resident 1968–70

Lin, K. Y. M.D.—Resident 1948

Lin, Shu-Ren M.D.—Associate
in Radiology 1972–73

Linnemann, Roger E. M.D.—
Associate in Radiology
1972–73

Littman, Philip M.D.—Resident
1972–73

Lockwood, Robert M. M.D.—
Resident 1949

Loigman, Barry I. M.D.—
Departmental Resident 1964

Lloyd, Herbert M. M.D.—
Departmental Resident
1964–66; Associate in
Radiology 1967

Lyon, James A. M.D.—Resident
1954; American Cancer Society
(Philadelphia Division) Fellow

1955; American Cancer Society
(National Organization) Fellow
1956

McClenahan, John M.D.—
Visiting Radiologist
1959–69

McLendon, Margaret—
Diagnostic Technician 1941

Mahoney, J. Francis M.D.—
Resident in Radiology
1942–44; Associate in
Radiology 1945–46

Malen, David S. M.D.—Resident
1947–49

Maltais, Roger M.D.—House
Staff 1961; American Cancer
Society (Philadelphia Division)
Fellow 1961

Manlio, Ferdinand L. D.O.—
Resident 1970–71

Marciniak, Roman M.D.—House
Staff 1960–61

Matasar, Kenneth W. M.D.—
Resident 1970–73

Mendelsohn, Mortimer M.D.,
Ph.D.—Radiobiologist
1958–62; Associate in
Radiology 1964–73 (no
information available to
determine title during 1963)

Miller, Alfred O. M.D.—
Resident 1946–48

Miller, Garrett R. M.D.—Fellow
in Roentgenology 1930; Fellow
in Radiology 1931–32

Miller, Harris P. M.D.—Resident
1972–73

Miller, Marlyn W. M.D.—
Resident 1947 and 1949

Miller, S. Thomas M.D.—Fellow in
Radiology 1942; Resident 1943

Miller, Wallace T. M.D.—House
Staff 1958–60; Trainee,
National Cancer Institute
1959–60; Associate in

Radiology 1961 and 1964–73 (no information available to determine status in 1963)

Mishkin, Mark M. M.D.—House Staff 1958–60; Trainee, National Cancer Institute 1959–60; Associate in Radiology 1961–73

Moraes, Cassio R. M.D.—Resident 1969–70

Muir, Mark W. M.D.—Resident 1950–51

Mulhern, Charles B. M.D.—Resident 1972–73

Munson, Frederick J. M.D.—House Staff 1957; Trainee, National Cancer Institute 1958–59; Visiting Radiologist 1960–61

Murray, Anne C.—Technician 1933–35; Secretary 1936

Nagle, Douglas B., Jr. M.D.—Resident 1947–49; Heublein Fellow 1950

Nagle, Sara C. R.N.—Diagnostic Technician 1936–41

Nagle, Walter W. M.D.—Resident 1951; DuPont Fellow 1953; Damon Runyon Fellow (American Cancer Society) 1954; Trainee, National Cancer Institute 1955

Neil, William H. M.D.—Resident 1954; Pennsylvania Manufacturers Association Fellow 1955

Nenninger, Robert H. M.D.—Resident 1970–73

Neuhauser, Edward B.D. M.D.—Resident and Assistant Instructor in Radiology 1940; Fellow and Assistant Instructor 1941; Fellow 1942

Newell, W. A. M.D.—Assistant Roentgenologist 1917–21

Noble, Paul R. M.D.—Resident 1947–49

Noel, Alice B. R.N.—Nurse and Technician 1925–26

Oberkircher, Paul E. M.D.—Associate in Radiology 1970–73

O'Hara, A. Edward M.D.—Resident 1950; DuPont Fellow 1951; Resident 1952, Pennsylvania Manufacturers Association Fellow 1954; Trainee, National Cancer Institute 1955

O'Neill, Dallett B. M.S.—Consultant Engineer 1940–41

Osgood, Ellis C. M.D.—Resident in Radiology 1942 and 1944

Osmond, Leslie H. M.D.—Fellow in Radiology 1933–34

Owsley, William C. M.D.—Resident 1950; Heublein Fellow 1951; Trainee, National Cancer Institute 1952

Palmer, Philip E. S. M.B.B.S.—Associate in Radiology 1970–71

Pancoast, Henry K. M.D.—Skiagrapher 1902–10; Professor of Roentgenology 1911; Roentgenologist and Professor of Roentgenology 1912–23; Chief of Roentgenology Clinic 1924–30; Professor of Radiology 1931–39

Patterson, Stuart D. M.D.—Resident 1948

Paysek, Edward J. M.D.—Resident 1955; American Cancer Society (Philadelphia Division) Fellow 1956; Trainee, National Cancer Institute 1957

Pendergrass, Eugene P. M.D.—Assistant Roentgenologist

1920–23; Assistant Chief of
Roentgenology Clinic 1924–27;
Assistant Chief of Clinic and
Associate in Roentgenology
1928–29; Assistant Chief of
Clinic and Assistant Professor
of Roentgenology 1930;
Assistant Professor of
Radiology 1931–36; Professor
of Radiology 1937–38; Chief
of Clinic 1939–61; Director of
Donner Center 1959–61; Vice
President of Diagnostic Clinic
1960; School of Nursing
Faculty 1960; Emeritus
Professor 1962 and 1964;
Emeritus Chief and Matthew
J. Wilson Professor in
Research Radiology 1965–66;
Emeritus Chief 1967–73

Pendergrass, Henry P. M.D.—
Resident 1954–56; Associate in
Radiology 1957–58 and 1961;
American Cancer Society
(National Organization) Fellow
1957

Perna, Francis M.D.—House
Staff 1962

Perritt, J. Olin, Jr. M.D.—
Resident 1954; DuPont Fellow
1955; Trainee, National Cancer
Institute 1956

Perryman, Charles R. M.D.—
Resident 1945; Associate in
Radiology 1946–49

Petrella, Edward J. M.D.—
Resident 1972–73

Phillips, John M. M.D.—
Resident 1949; American
Cancer Society (Philadelphia
Division) Fellow 1950–51

Pitol, Adan M.D.—Resident
1953; Heublein Fellow 1954;
DuPont Fellow 1954

Polutan, Rustico C. M.D.—

Resident 1972–73

Post, Lawrence A. M.D.—
Resident 1954; Trainee,
National Cancer Institute
1955–56

Powell, Clinton C. M.D.—
Resident 1953–54

Press, Harry C. M.D.—
Departmental Resident
1964–65

Pryde, Arthur W. M.D.—
Resident 1946–48

Pryor, T. Hunter M.D.—DuPont
Fellow 1957; Trainee, National
Cancer Institute 1958–59;
Associate in Radiology 1959

Raphael, Robert L. M.D.—
Resident 1950; Pennsylvania
Manufacturers Association
Fellow 1951–52

Rathbone, Ralph Rhett, M.D.—
Fellow in Radiology (Resident)
1932; Fellow in Radiology
1933

Raventos, Antolin M.D.—
Associate in Radiology
1954–70; School of Nursing
Faculty 1958–61

Reeves, John D. M.D.—Resident
1952–53

Ripple, Richard C. M.D.—
Resident 1947–49; Trainee,
National Cancer Institute
1950, Resident 1951

Ritchie, David M.D.—House
Staff 1958–61; American
Cancer Society Fellow 1959;
Trainee, National Cancer
Institute 1960; DuPont Fellow
1961

Rittenberg, Gerald M. M.D.—
Resident 1968–71

Ritter, Vern W. M.D.—Resident
1947; Trainee, National Cancer
Institute 1948; Resident 1949–50

Roberts, Agrippa G. M.D.—
Resident in Radiology 1942,
1944, 1946–47

Rockoff, S. David M.D.—House
Staff 1959–61; Trainee,
National Cancer Institute
1959–61

Rosenkrantz, Harvey M.D.—
Resident 1972–73

Rothenberg, Howard P. M.D.—
Resident 1970–73

Rozen, Jay I. M.D.—
Departmental Resident
1965–69

Ryan, Richard R. M.D.—
Associate in Radiology
1968–69

Salner, Nathan P. M.D.—
Resident 1945–46; Visiting
Staff 1950–52; Associate in
Radiology 1953–56; Visiting
Radiologist 1966–71

Sanders, Theodore P. M.D.—
Departmental Resident
1964–66; Associate in
Radiology 1967–73

Sathaphatayavongs, Boonchuey
M.D.—Resident 1970–73

Schapiro, Rolf L. M.D.—
Resident 1966–69

Schilling, Marie A. R.N.—Nurse
Technician 1929–30

Scholl, Harvey W. M.D.—
Resident 1969–73

Schor, George E. M.D.—Resident
1971–73

Schreiber, Michael N. M.D.—
Resident 1971–73

Schwade, James R. M.D.—
Resident 1972–73

Schwartz, Armin M.D.—
Visiting Fellow in Radiology
1954

Scott, John R. M.D.—Resident
1968–71

Scott, Horace M.D.—House Staff
1959–61; Trainee, National
Cancer Institute 1960;
Pennsylvania Manufacturers
Association Fellow 1961

Seal, Sam H. M.D.—Resident
1950–51

Sedlak, Stephen P. M.D.—
Pennsylvania Manufacturers
Association Fellow 1953;
Trainee, National Cancer
Institute 1954

Shah, Sudhir H. M.B., B.S.—
Resident 1968–69

Shapeero, Lorraine G. M.D.—
Resident 1971–73

Shiffer, Paul H. M.D.—Resident
1947; Visiting Radiologist
1959–64

Shuman, Hind M.D.—House
Staff 1962; American Cancer
Society (National
Organization) Fellow 1962;
Departmental Resident 1964

Siu, Marc K. P. M.D.—Resident
1949

Smith, Hugh P. M.D.—Resident
1950–51

Smyth, Murray G., Jr. M.D.—
Research Fellow in Isotopes
1954–55

Somburanasin, Racha M.D.—
Resident 1970–71

Stephenson, David J. M.D.—
Resident 1953–54; American
Cancer Society (Philadelphia
Division) Fellow 1955;
Pennsylvania Manufacturers
Association Fellow 1956

Stolz, Jonathan L. M.D.—
Resident 1971–73

Suh, Chul Sung M.D.—Resident
1956; Hueblein Fellow 1958

Sullivan, Michael A. M.D.—
Resident 1966–69

Sundaravej, Kundala M.D.—
Heublein Fellow 1957–58

Talley, Danniel D. III M.D.—
Resident 1949; DuPont Fellow
1950; Pennsylvania
Manufacturers Association
Fellow 1950–51

Thomas, Sydney F. M.D.—
Associate in Radiology 1962

Thorner, Rosalind S. M.D.—
Fellow in Radiology 1938;
Assistant Instructor in
Radiology 1939–40

Thorwarth, William T. M.D.—
Resident 1955; DuPont Fellow
1956; Trainee, National Cancer
Institute 1957; Visiting
Radiologist 1965–73

Timmermans, Winand M.D.—
House Staff 1960–61

Tomsula, Joseph P. M.D.—
Resident 1947; Trainee,
National Cancer Institute
1948

Tondreau, Roderick L. M.D.—
Associate in Radiology
1952–58

Toth, Steven M.D.—House Staff
1962; University of
Pennsylvania Radiology Fund
Fellow 1962; Departmental
Resident 1964; Associate in
Radiology 1966–67

Townsend, DeWayne M.D.—
Resident 1944

Tristan, Theodore A. M.D.—
Resident 1954; American
Cancer Society (New York
Division) Fellow 1955;
American Cancer Society
(National Organization) Fellow
1956; Associate in Radiology
1960–66

Tuddenham, William J. M.D.—
Resident 1952; A. Atwater

Kent Fellow 1953; Trainee,
National Cancer Institute
1954–55; Associate in
Radiology 1955–58 and 1962;
Pennsylvania Manufacturers
Association Fellow 1955; James
Picker Scholar in Radiologic
Research 1957; Diagnostic
Division and Associate
Professor Radiology 1959–61;
Assistant Director of Donner
Center 1959–61; Visiting
Radiologist 1966–73

Urso, May G. M.D.—Resident
1970

Van der Walt, Marthinus J.
M.D.—Resident 1952;
Heublein Fellow 1953

Viamonte, Manuel, Jr. M.D.—
House Staff 1957; American
Cancer Society (National
Organization) Fellow 1958

Warden, John S. M.D.—Resident
1956; Trainee, National Cancer
Institute 1957–58;
Pennsylvania Manufacturers
Association Fellow 1957

Warren, S. Reid, Jr. Sc.D.—
Consultant Engineer 1940–41;
Consultant Physicist 1943–73

Wartella, Stephen, Jr. M.D.—
Resident 1953–55

Wehl, Charles M. M.S.—
Consultant Engineer 1940–41

Weigen, John F. M.D.—Resident
1949; Trainee, National Cancer
Institute 1950–52

Weigensberg, Irving M.D.—
House Staff 1961–62; Trainee,
National Cancer Institute
1962; Departmental Resident
1964

Wendle, Lida V. R.N.—
Diagnostic Technician 1937–39

White, Francis A. M.D.—

Resident 1956; American Cancer Society (National Organization) Fellow 1957; Trainee, National Cancer Institute 1958; DuPont Fellow 1958

White, Lucy G. R.N.—Nurse Technician 1929–30

Williams, Burton L. M.D.— Associate in Radiology 1969–73

Wilson, Richard V. M.D.— Resident 1951; Trainee, National Cancer Institute 1952–53

Winston, Joseph P. M.D.— House Staff 1958–60; American Cancer Society Fellow 1959–60; School of Nursing Faculty 1959 and 1961; Associate in Radiology 1961; Visiting Radiologist 1962–71

Winston, Norman J. M.D.— Resident 1951; Trainee, National Cancer Institute 1952

Wise, Helen A. R.N.— Roentgenology, Nurse in Charge 1924; Nurse and Technician 1925–26

Wolfman, Harvey T. M.D.— Resident 1971–73

Woods, Ruth Riegel R.N.— Nurse Technician 1931; Technician 1932–33

Yood, Norman L. M.D.— Resident 1954

Zarembok, Irwin M.D.— Resident 1970, 1972–73

Zatz, Leslie M. M.D.—Resident 1956; American Cancer Society (National Organization) Fellow 1957; House Staff 1958

Zeiger, Louis S. M.D.—Resident 1971

Zimmerman, Norval F. M.D.— Resident 1949; Heublein Fellow 1950–51; Pennsylvania Manufacturers Association Fellow 1952

Zimmerman, Robert A. M.D.— Resident 1966–69; Associate in Radiology 1972–73

Zirkle, Raymond E. A.B., Ph.D. —Consultant Bio-Physicist 1938–39

Bibliography

Air Hygiene Foundation of America, Inc. *The Comparative Values of Chest Roentgenograms Made on Film and on Paper for Industrial Surveys.* Medical Series, Bulletin No. II. Pittsburgh: Air Hygiene Foundation of America, Inc., 1939.

American Roentgen Ray Society. *Transactions of the Fourth Annual Meeting of the American Roentgen Ray Society, December 9–10, 1903.* Philadelphia: 1904.

Association of Pendergrass Fellows. *Grassroots, the Official Organ of the Association of Pendergrass Fellows.* Philadelphia.

Brown, Percy. *American Martyrs to Science through the Roentgen Rays.* Springfield, Illinois: Charles C. Thomas, 1936.

———. "Henry Khunrath Pancoast—An Appreciation." *The American Journal of Roentgenology and Radium Therapy* **38** (1937): 4–10.

Cheyney, Edward Potts. *History of the University of Pennsylvania, 1740–1940.* Philadelphia: University of Pennsylvania Press, 1940.

Corner, George W. *Two Centuries of Medicine: A History of the School of Medicine, University of Pennsylvania.* Philadelphia: J. B. Lippincott Company, 1965.

Department of Radiology Staff Physicians, Hospital of the University of Pennsylvania. *Meeting Minutes,* July, 1942 through September, 1962.

Department of Radiology Staff Technicians and Secretaries, Hospital of the University of Pennsylvania. *Meeting Minutes,* February, 1951 through May, 1956.

Dowlin, Cornell M., ed. *The University of Pennsylvania Today, Its Buildings, Departments and Work.* Philadelphia: University of Pennsylvania Press, 1940.

Evans, William A. "American Pioneers in Radiology." In *The Science of Radiology,* edited by Otto Glasser, pp. 22–38. Springfield, Illinois: Charles C. Thomas, 1933.

Fuchs, Arthur W. "Radiographic Recording Media and Screens." In *The*

Science of Radiology, edited by Otto Glasser, pp. 97–119. Springfield, Illinois: Charles C. Thomas, 1933.

Goodspeed, Arthur W. "Remarks made at the Demonstration of the Röntgen Ray, at Stated Meeting, February 21, 1896." *Proceedings of The American Philosophical Society* **35** (1896): 16–36.

Hendricks, Gordon. *Eadweard Muybridge: The Father of the Motion Picture.* New York: Grossman Publishers, 1975.

"Henry Khunrath Pancoast." *Radiology and Clinical Photography* **15** (1939).

Holmes, George W. "American Radiology: Its Contributions to the Diagnosis and Treatment of Disease." *Journal of the American Medical Association* **135** (1947): 327–30.

Hospital of the University of Pennsylvania. *Annual Report of the Board of Managers* (1899–1963) and *Annual Report* (1964–1973). Philadelphia.

Leonard, Charles Lester. "The Application of the Roentgen Rays to Medical Diagnosis." *Journal of the American Medical Association* **29** (1897): 1157–58.

————. "The Diagnosis of Calculus Nephritis by Means of the Roentgen Rays." *The Philadelphia Medical Journal* **II** (1898): 388–90.

————. "A Double Focus X-ray Tube for the Accurate Localization by Fluoroscope or Photographic Plate of Foreign Bodies." *The American X-ray Journal* **5** (1899): 659–62.

————. "The Influence of the X-ray Method of Diagnosis upon the Treatment of Fractures." *Therapeutic Gazette* **14** (1898): 177–9.

————. "Methods of Precision in Locating Foreign Bodies in the Head by Means of the Roentgen Rays, with Special Reference to Foreign Bodies in the Eye." *Annals of Ophthalmology* **7** (1898): 161–70.

Pancoast, Henry K. "Reminiscences of a Radiologist." *American Journal of Roentgenology and Radium Therapy* **39** (1938): 169–86.

Pendergrass, Eugene P. and Barden, Robert P. "Radiological Service Advanced by Design." *Modern Hospital* **60** (1943): 68–70.

Pendergrass, Eugene P., Warren, S. Reid, and Haagensen, D. E. *A Comparison of Stereoscopic Miniature Chest Films, Single Roentgenograms on Paper, and Single Roentgenograms on Large Films.* Medical Series, Bulletin No. V. Pittsburgh: Industrial Hygiene Foundation of America, Inc., 1942.

Pfahler, George E. "The Early History of Roentgenology in Philadelphia: The History of the Philadelphia Roentgen Ray Society, Part I: 1899–1920." *American Journal of Roentgenology, Radium Therapy and Nuclear Medicine* **75** (1956): 14–22.

Philadelphia. Department of Radiology. Hospital of the University of Pennsylvania. Interne's Register, September 1933 through August 1948.

————. Department of Radiology. Hospital of the University of Pennsylvania. Records and Registers. Donner Center.

————. Department of Radiology. Hospital of the University of Pennsylvania. Records and Registers. Miscellaneous Papers.

_____. Department of Radiology. Hospital of the University of Pennsylvania. Records and Registers. Pendergrass Fellows.

_____. Department of Radiology. Hospital of the University of Pennsylvania. Research Files. Donner Center and Foundation.

_____. Hospital of the University of Pennsylvania. Documents. Document Box.

_____. Moore School of Electrical Engineering. University of Pennsylvania. Research Files. "Notes on Electromedical Work in the Moore School of Electrical Engineering, 24 July 1964" [by S. Reid Warren, Jr.].

_____. University of Pennsylvania Archives. Medico-Chirurgical College, *Trustee Minutes.*

Richards, Horace C. "Arthur Willis Goodspeed: An Obituary." *American Philosophical Society Yearbook, 1943.* Philadelphia: 1944.

Stephenson, Mary Virginia. *The First Fifty Years of the Training School for Nurses of the Hospital of the University of Pennsylvania.* Philadelphia: J. B. Lippincott Company, 1940.

University of Pennsylvania. *Board of Trustees Minutes.* Volume 15 (1911), Volume 20 (1930).

_____. *Catalogue of the University of Pennsylvania, Fasciculus of the Department of Medicine.* Philadelphia.

_____. *Scope, 1910; University of Pennsylvania Yearbook: School of Medicine.* Philadelphia: 1910.

_____. *The University Bulletin: Graduate School of Medicine, 1919–20.* Philadelphia: 1919.

_____. *University of Pennsylvania Bulletin: School of Medicine,* **77** (1977–78). Philadelphia: 1976.

_____. *University of Pennsylvania Medical Center Annual Report, 1970–71.* Philadelphia: 1971.

_____. *University of Pennsylvania Medical Center Biennial Report, 1971–73.* Philadelphia: 1973.

_____. *University of Pennsylvania Medical Center Triennial Report, 1973–76.* Philadelphia: 1976.

White, J. William. "A Foreign Body in the Esophagus Detected and Located by Röntgen Rays." *University Medical Magazine* **8** (1896): 710–15.

White, J. William, Goodspeed, Arthur W., and Leonard, Charles L. "Cases Illustrative of the Practical Application of the Röntgen Rays in Surgery." *American Journal of the Medical Sciences* **112** (1896): 125–47.

Willard, DeForest. "History and Description of the D. Haynes Agnew Memorial Pavilion of the University Hospital." In *The Opening of the Agnew Wing at the Hospital of the University of Pennsylvania, October 15, 1897.* Philadelphia: J. B. Lippincott Company, 1897.

"The Wilson Professorship." *Medical Affairs* **II** (1961): 28–9.

Full-Time Faculty, 1981

Department of Radiology
Hospital of the University of Pennsylvania

ADMINISTRATION

Stanley Baum, M.D., Eugene P. Pendergrass Professor of Radiology, Chairman
Wallace T. Miller, M.D., Professor of Radiology, Vice Chairman
Ronald L. Arenson, M.D., Associate Professor of Radiology, Director of Administrative Services

SPECIALTIES

ANGIO-
GRAPHY
Stanley Baum, M.D., Professor of Radiology
David B. Freiman, M.D., Assistant Professor of Radiology
Gordon K. McLean, M.D., Assistant Professor of Radiology
Ernest J. Ring, M.D., Professor of Radiology (Chief)
Gerald L. Wolf, M.D., Professor of Radiology

GI SECTION
Hans Herlinger, M.D., Professor of Radiology
Herbert Y. Kressel, M.D., Associate Professor of Radiology
Igor Laufer, M.D., Professor of Radiology (Chief)

[161]

GU SECTION   Marc P. Banner, M.D., Associate Professor of
Radiology

Howard M. Pollack, M.D., Professor of Radiology
(Chief)

OUT PATIENT   Adele K. Friedman, M.D., Associate Professor of
Radiology (Chief)

Rosalind H. Troupin, M.D., Professor of
Radiology

NEURO-
RADIOLOGY   Larissa T. Bilaniuk, M.D., Associate Professor of
Radiology

Herbert I. Goldberg, M.D., Professor of Radiology

Robert I. Grossman, M.D., Assistant Professor of
Radiology

Robert A. Zimmerman, M.D., Professor of
Radiology (Chief)

NUCLEAR
MEDICINE   Abass Alavi, M.D., Associate Professor of
Radiology (Chief)

Michael J. Eymontt, M.D., Assistant Professor of
Radiology

P. Todd Makler, Jr., M.D., Assistant Professor of
Radiology

Gerd Muehllehner, Ph.D., Associate Professor of
Radiology

Muni M. Staum, Ph.D., Research Specialist

ORTHO-
PAEDIC
SECTION   John A. Bonavita, M.D., Assistant Professor of
Radiology

Murray K. Dalinka, M.D., Professor of Radiology
(Chief)

Morrison E. Kricun, M.D., Associate Professor of
Radiology

VA-
DIAGNOSTIC   Vijay K. Gohel, M.D., Associate Professor of
Radiology (Chief)

David M. Rogovitz, M.D., Assistant Professor of
Radiology

Jay S. Rosenblum, M.D., Assistant Professor of
Radiology

Arlyne T. Shockman, M.D., Associate Professor of
Radiology

PULMON-ARY/ CHEST	David M. Epstein, M.D., Assistant Professor of Radiology Warren B. Gefter, M.D., Assistant Professor of Radiology Wallace T. Miller, M.D., Professor of Radiology (Chief)
US/CT	Ronald L. Arenson, M.D., Associate Professor of Radiology Peter H. Arger, M.D., Professor of Radiology (Chief) Leon Axel, Ph.D., M.D., Assistant Professor of Radiology Richard L. Baron, M.D., Assistant Professor of Radiology Beverly G. Coleman, M.D., Assistant Professor of Radiology
RESEARCH	Gabor T. Herman, Ph.D., Professor of Radiology Harold L. Kundel, M.D., Professor of Radiology (Chief) Robert LeVeen, M.D., Assistant Professor of Radiology Robert M. Lewitt, Ph.D., Research Assistant Professor of Radiology Heang Kim Tuy, Ph.D., Research Assistant Professor of Radiology Jack W. London, Ph.D., Assistant Professor of Radiology
VA-NUCLEAR MEDICINE	Harold A. Goldstein, M.D., Assistant Professor of Radiology John R. Hansell, M.D., Associate Professor of Radiology (Chief)
RADIO-LOGICAL PHYSICS	John Hale, Ph.D., Professor of Radiology